Nutrients for Neuropathy

Nutrients for Neuropathy

(Volume 3 in the Numb Toes Series)

By

John A. Senneff

MEDPRESS
San Antonio, Texas

© 2002 by John A. Senneff

Published by
MedPress
P.O. Box 691546
San Antonio, TX 78269
www.medpress.com

Library of Congress Control Number: 2002106050

ISBN: 0-9671107-5-0

This text is printed on acid-free paper.

Printed in the United States of America.

10   9   8   7   6   5   4   3   2   1

*To those doctors willing to suggest that
nutritional approaches may sometimes be preferred
to a total regime of prescription medications*

Contents

Foreword to the Foreword

Dr. Laurence Kinsella, author of the Foreword to this book, has been closely identified with nutrients and their implications for peripheral neuropathy for many years. He is widely recognized as an authority on these matters throughout the world. I am grateful he consented to review my book, making a number of helpful suggestions in the process, and was willing to write the Foreword.

Dr. Kinsella has independently authored numerous articles and book chapters, co-authored many studies and talked extensively on a number of the matters dealt with in this book. In August 2001, for example, he presented a major lecture, "Nutrition and Neuropathy," in Rome, Italy, to a distinguished gathering of neurologists from all over the world.

Currently Dr. Kinsella is the Director of the Neurophysiology Laboratory at the Tenet-Forest Park Hospital in St. Louis, Missouri, as well as Associate Professor of Neurology at the St. Louis University School of Medicine. Before that he was the Chief of the Division of Neurology at the Mt. Sinai Medical Center. Earlier neurology posts were at Case Western Reserve University in Cleveland, Ohio, Columbia University in New York City, and Brown University in Providence, Rhode Island.

Foreword

I was delighted to have the opportunity to write a brief Foreword for John's new book. This is his third treatise on a topic that has been all too often ignored in the lay press. For those who suffer from peripheral neuropathy, his books have been a comfort and a welcomed relief.

"Numb Toes and Aching Soles" and "Numb Toes and Other Woes," introduced the topic of peripheral neuropathy, its causes, and standard as well as alternative treatments. John now moves into the more treacherous task of weighing often conflicting evidence on the usefulness of dietary and nutritional supplements for neuropathy.

There are a number of nutrients that are necessary for normal nerve growth. Deficiencies of these vitamins may lead to nerve injury. These include thiamine (B1), cobalamin (B12), and pyridoxine (B6). Other nutrients required for normal nerve growth are lipids, glucose, and protein.

It would be nice to know the answer to the following questions: (1) What nutrients does the peripheral nerve need? (2) What nutrients are potentially harmful? (3) Are any supplements proven to enhance nerve function?

What Nutrients Does the Peripheral Nerve Need?

Thiamine, cobalamin, and pyridoxine, as well as glucose, protein, lipids, oxygen, and growth factors are necessary for normal nerve function. Much of what we know about the function of nutrients comes from studying their deficiency states, particularly in the case of thiamine which causes beriberi; vitamin B12 deficiency which causes dysfunction of the spinal cord and peripheral nerves and anemia; and pyridoxine deficiency which may also cause nerve injury.

What Nutrients Are Potentially Harmful?

There are a number of nutrients that have been determined to be harmful, not only to the peripheral nerves, but also to the nervous system in general. These include megadose pyridoxine in excess of 200 mg daily. Pyridoxine is unique in that both an excess and a deficiency cause injury to the peripheral nervous system. Pyridoxine is an exception to the commonly held misconception that megadose B complex vitamins cannot hurt you because they are excreted in the urine.

Another potential cause of harm are Chinese herbal remedies. Many of these contain arsenic, lead, and mercury, and there have been several cases of arsenic neuropathy documented in patients who had been using Chinese herbal remedies.

St. John's Wort, when boiled in large quantities from the root, may cause severe photosensitivity and a burning neuropathic pain on sun-exposed areas. Gingko biloba has been known to cause hemorrhage in the brain. Many weight loss remedies contain ephedra, a naturally occurring form of adrenaline. This substance has been associated with heart attack and stroke and should be avoided.

Are Any Supplements Proven to Enhance Nerve Function?

As John's book indicates, there is reasonably good evidence that, in addition to some of the vitamins in the B complex, certain nutrients such as alpha-lipoic acid (ALA), gamma linolenic acid (GLA), and three or four minerals, contribute to nerve health and may in certain cases help in the management of peripheral neuropathy.

However, it is also true, as he points out, that there are too few scientifically based studies of long-term duration to draw long-term conclusions on these matters. In this regard the best studies that give the most reliable data are double blind, randomized, controlled trials, meaning that neither the patient nor the doctor knows whether the individual is receiving or not receiving the particular supplement in question. A standardized measurement of nerve function is performed and at the end of the trial, the blinding is removed, and the data are available for review to see whether or not the dietary supplement was of any benefit. These types of studies are expensive and difficult to do and, as mentioned in John's book, are not subsidized by drug companies in this country since it is not possible to patent most dietary supplements.

Nevertheless, *Nutrients for Neuropathy* succeeds in bringing together a great deal of important information on nutrients. John's treatment of dietary supplements is comprehensive and should prove valuable for those who are afflicted with peripheral neuropathy.

Laurence J. Kinsella, M.D.
St. Louis, Missouri

Introduction

This book is intended for those PNers[1] who are fed up with medications that don't work, that are costly, and that sometimes have appalling side effects. I believe there is another, better answer for most of us, namely **nutrient supplements**. These vitamins, minerals and related substances added to our diets may not entirely eliminate our need for medications (though in some cases they could), but they surely can help reduce our total reliance on drugs.

To put this in perspective, there is **no prescription drug** currently available to **cure** peripheral neuropathy. (If there were one at a reasonable cost and with minimal

---

[1] PNers is the name I gave in my first book—*Numb Toes and Aching Soles: Coping with Peripheral Neuropathy* (MedPress 1999)—to those of us who have this obnoxious malady. That book will hereinafter be referred to as *Toes and Soles*. My second book, *Numb Toes and Other Woes: More on Peripheral Neuropathy* (MedPress 2001), which updates that information, will be referred to as *Toes and Woes*. If you are stuck with PN, or have symptoms such as aching, burning pains in your feet, or foot or toe numbness, tingling in your hands, or muscular weakness that is causing you problems, all of which strongly suggest the possibility of peripheral neuropathy, you definitely need to educate yourself. That is the purpose of those two books. Besides, this book won't make nearly as much sense to you if you haven't read them! (Order forms for *Toes and Soles* and *Toes and Woes* are at the back of this book.)

side effects there would be little need for a book such as this, though there might still be a place for a book on the use of supplements for helping to **prevent** PN.)

In fact as of the time this was written there were only two drugs specifically approved by the Food and Drug Administration—the arbiter of such matters—to even **deal** with peripheral neuropathy. Each was originally designed to treat specialized forms of the disorder: carbamazepine (trade name Tegretol), an anticonvulsant, was developed to cope with trigeminal neuralgia, a facial nerve pain syndrome. Lidoderm, a transdermal (meaning absorbed through the skin) formulation of lidocaine, was intended for postherpetic neuralgia, a type of neuropathic pain sometimes associated with shingles. (They both have broader neuropathic applications now.) Other drugs being prescribed today for PN were originally approved for other ailments. The FDA has informally permitted these **"off label"** uses in treating peripheral neuropathy as a matter of policy. (According to an FDA spokesman, although physicians may prescribe drugs for uses that are different from those approved, representatives of drug companies are not allowed to market or promote these off-label uses.)

Toes and Soles and *Toes and Woes* discuss these various pharmaceuticals in some detail. In almost every instance they are directed to **pain** or other **symptomatic relief**.[2] There are few medications offering hope of **repairing** the

---

[2] An excellent article on pain appeared in the December 16, 2001, issue of *The New York Times*. The work of Dr. Daniel Carr at the New England Pain Center in Boston was discussed at length. In dealing

nerves or their myelin coating and **restoring** neural function so that **long-term** relief can be anticipated.[3]

Even considering the rather modest goals of symptomatic relief set for these drugs in dealing with PN, there are several problems with which they must contend. First, no one can be sure which of the two dozen or so is going to work (if any at all) for a particular individual. It is often a matter of lengthy trial and error to find a medication that will help. In the meanwhile the patient goes on suffering, being told that he or she needs to give whatever drug is prescribed "enough time to do its job," even if that means weeks of possible agony until the next one is tried.[4]

---

with pain as a disease itself which requires treating—and not just a symptom of something else—Dr. Carr is trying to find the "master gene switch" which might turn pain "off."

[3] A couple of the immunosuppressants mentioned in *Toes and Soles* and *Toes and Woes* appear to offer at least short term benefits with respect to nerve re-myelination, but there is a risk of possibly debilitating side effects such as gastritis, tremors, and glaucoma.

Other drugs are in the wings, though, which may truly offer more than just symptomatic relief. Note the following comment which appeared in a recent story concerning the corporate merger between Bio-Technology General and Myelos Corporation:

> "Prosaptide was shown to not only alleviate peripheral neuropathic pain but also to *reverse the underlying neuropathy*, thereby inducing neuronal regeneration and preventing neuronal death. The data from these studies strongly suggest that if these findings are replicated in human clinical trials, there may well be additional potential for Prosaptide in the treatment of diabetic peripheral neuropathy, *over and above its demonstrated ability to decrease neuropathic pain*. No approved drugs are available to prevent or reverse the neuropathy itself. [Emphases added]" As of the time this was written, Prosaptide was scheduled for Phase II (b) studies, according to Bio-Technology General.

[4] *Toes and Woes* noted a somber view concerning pain relief via conventional medicine in quoting Professor Clifford J. Woolf of the

Also—let's face it—many doctors, well-meaning though they be, are just not up to speed in treating an ailment as challenging as PN. They may not know about the various treatment possibilities such as nutrient supplementation, and they may feel themselves too busy to stay current and try other approaches, particularly when they may secretly suspect that the problem is in the patient's head rather than his or her feet, hands, legs, or arms or wherever the patient, in fact, happens to hurt.[5]

Harvard Medical School, writing on "Neuropathic Pain: Aetiology, Symptoms, Mechanisms, and Management":

> "[P]harmacotherapy for neuropathic pain has been disappointing. Patients with neuropathic pain do not respond to non-steroidal anti-inflammatory drugs and resistance or insensitivity to opiates is common. Patients are usually treated empirically with tricyclic or serotonin and norepinephrine uptake inhibitors, antidepressants, and anticonvulsants that all have limited efficacy and undesirable side-effects. Neurosurgical lesions have a neglible role and functional neurosurgery, including dorsal column or brain stimulation, is controversial, although transcutaneous nerve stimulation may provide some relief. Local anaesthetic blocks targeted at trigger points, peripheral nerves, plexi, dorsal roots, and the sympathetic nervous system have useful but short-lived effects; longer lasting blocks by phenol injection or cryotherapy risk irreversible functional impairment and have not been tested in placebo-controlled trials. . . . There is no treatment to prevent the development of neuropathic pain, nor to adequately, predictably, and specifically control established neuropathic pain." *Lancet* (1999; 353: 959–64).

Following this quote I said that his views, though perhaps unnecessarily grim, make the case even stronger for the implementation of nutrient strategies. Time has only increased my belief in that regard—hence this book.

[5] I think the following observation from the Chromium Information Bureau is interesting—and cogent—in regard to why many doctors may not be recommending supplements:

> "The marketing of nutritional therapies to physicians and other health professionals is not nearly as extensive as pharmaceutical marketing; since profits from nutritional therapies are significantly smaller than those from pharmaceuticals, supplement manufacturers

And as for those **side effects**—whoo! Depending on the particular drug, they can include dizziness, insomnia, mental lapses, headaches, blurred vision, rashes, internal bleeding, constipation, hypotension or hepatitis. Certainly not everyone suffers such consequences, but they occur often enough to make one cautious about using these medications. Read about a few of the patient treatment experiences in *Toes and Soles* or on Internet bulletin boards. Some of them describe side effects that seem almost worse than the neuropathy itself!

On the other hand, troublesome or dangerous side effects are rather infrequent with most nutrients unless massive doses are taken.[6] (A side note here: Some medical

---

cannot justify the large capital outlays needed for the promotional and educational materials for physicians. In addition, representatives of drug manufacturers frequently call on physicians to present them with new research data and samples of their products. Direct mail and advertising are other means by which pharmaceutical manufacturers get important information about their products to doctors. The same promotional and educational budgets are not available in the nutritional area."

[6] A study reported in the October 23, 2000, issue of the eMedicine Journal (Volume 2, Number 10), concerning acute or chronic overdoses, reported that of 40,000 "exposures," which I assume meant reported incidents, there were eight "major adverse outcomes" and one death. Another study indicated that there were 2556 fatalities due to drug overdoses from 1983 to 1990 compared with no fatalities due to high doses of vitamin supplements.

As I write these very words, the following is on the front page of the *Wall Street Journal* (1/19/2002):

"Bayer said the number of deaths with a possible link to its Lipobay anticholesterol drug, marketed in the U.S. as Baycol, has risen to about 100, nearly double the previous estimate."

This concerning a drug which presumably had been thoroughly tested for safety as well as efficacy. The obvious message: Buyer beware of Bayer's Baycol.

professionals argue against the use of almost any supplement as being both unnecessary and possibly dangerous without making any distinctions among classes of nutrients. In the latter respect they usually point to instances where certain herbal products have caused health problems. Sometimes these problems were due to the careless way the products were manufactured or compounded and sometimes they were caused by interactions with prescription drugs—interactions, incidentally, which are generally predictable based on the pharmacological properties of the herb. The press then tends to pick up on these reports and follows the lead they have been given, carelessly putting all supplements in the same "things-to-be-avoided" category and scaring everybody in the process. That is truly a shame because there is ample authority and experience as to the safe use of the nutrients discussed in this book where used in the appropriate amounts.)

Of course **nutrient toxicity** can occur—as is true with taking too much of anything normally not harmful—and one needs to be aware of **maximum safe levels** as well as **drug interactions**. (Where information was available, toxicity and interactions are dealt with in the following chapters in connection with each of the various supplements discussed.) For these reasons, and because we are all individuals with differing **physiological** and **biological** make-ups,[7] it would be advisable to discuss with

---

[7] "Large differences in individual susceptibility to vitamin neurotoxicity probably exist." *Molecular Neurobiology* (1992 Spring; 6 (1): 41–73).

your doctor exactly what supplements you intend to use before embarking on a nutrient program.

As you will see from the studies reported in this book, in addition to short-term pain and other symptomatic relief, nutrients (and by extension nutrient supplements) offer at least the *possibility* of long-term, beneficial physiological and biological changes. These include the potential repair of nerves and their coatings and the restoration of neural function.[8]

Note that I stressed the word *possibility*. All that can be reasonably said at the current time, based on the studies and other information reported in this book, is that there is a decent chance certain nutrients, when administered in the correct dosages for a sufficient period, will produce an enduring neurological benefit in addition to short-term symptomatic improvement. There is a problem in substantiating **continuing** benefits, however; even though there is a growing mound of clinical studies showing the value of nutrient supplementation in treating peripheral neuropathy, there simply are not enough *long-term* investigations to prove *long-term* benefits. The paucity of multi-year studies is particularly evident in this country. Here there is no patent protection for vitamins, minerals and most other nutritional products and accordingly no particular incentives for companies to bear the costs of lengthy, expensive studies.

---

[8] Occasionally medical professionals use the following terms to explain the difference in treatments: "active treatment" or "specific therapy" is directed to the cure of a disease. "Palliative treatment" or "symptomatic therapy" is designed just for the relief of symptoms.

In this regard it is interesting to note in which countries most of the clinical studies for medications have been performed versus which countries nutrient studies have been conducted. You will see from *Toes and Soles* and *Toes and Woes* that practically all of the reported **medicine investigations** were accomplished in the United States. Here the **pharmaceutical companies** are the main sponsors of such studies inasmuch as they directly benefit from the proprietary protections the patent laws afford. Compare where the **nutrient studies** were performed; just about all were in countries such as Germany or France or Italy or Japan, countries where the **governments** have a long history of supporting nutrient investigations at their publics' expense and countries where supplements are part of mainstream medical practice.

The ideas for specific supplementations in the following chapters in general are based on **clinical studies** concerning **efficacy** of the various nutrients discussed as well as **appropriate dosages**. Unless there was **scientific evidence** that a particular supplement will or might produce a beneficial result for peripheral neuropathy or there was a long history of extensive use for that purpose with satisfactory outcomes, it was not included in these pages. You will see, though, in some instances there are conflicting views on the value of certain substances based on study conclusions that go in different directions. I have laid all this information out—in fact everything I could find in clinical studies and in "the literature"—so that you can see the whole picture for yourself.

The suggestions contained in the last chapter are based on my own assessment of these matters. Keep in mind, as those who have read *Toes and Soles* and *Toes and Woes* know, I am not a doctor treating peripheral neuropathy, just a retired lawyer afflicted with it like most of you who are reading this. As I wrote in the Preface to *Toes and Soles*, I consider that an advantage. I am not boxed in by any particular view because of prior training and can reach conclusions for myself based on the weight of the evidence as I see it (that's the lawyer in me talking).

As I stressed in my other two books on this subject and emphasize here, you ought to find a *qualified* physician with whom to work. Make sure he or she is one who understands and appreciates the value of nutrient supplementation in appropriate cases. Discuss with this doctor then the ideas presented here as they relate to your own situation.[9] Miriam Wetzel, Ph.D., Harvard Medical School, offers the following suggestions if you are looking for such a physician:

---

[9] The following idea was expressed by Jack Challem in a *Let's Live* magazine article a few years ago. Challem is the editor of *The Nutrition Reporter* and one of the leading nutrition writers in America, with published articles in *Modern Maturity*, the *Saturday Evening Post* and in many health magazines. What he wrote rather expresses my own thinking:

"While I believe everyone has an inalienable right to treat themselves, it's always best to work with a physician when treating a specific disease. At the very least, read up on the subject-public libraries, bookstores, and health food stores carry many health books."

What he said about reading books is particularly important for PNers because of the lack of understanding on the part of many medical professionals concerning our ailment. *We must educate ourselves!*

Check out the doctor's attitude toward complementary and alternative medicine. Talk to the doctor on the phone for five or 10 minutes. Have your questions ready and make notes. Pay attention to the quality of your discussion. Does it inspire your confidence? Consider whether you prefer a doctor who will take charge of your care, or one who will give you information and include you in making decisions.

Next, consider arranging an interview. Some doctors allow a 10- or 15-minute initial visit at no charge, but others don't. Instead, you may want to schedule a routine visit. During your visit, ask the doctor if he or she is familiar with complementary and alternative therapies.

Do not be reluctant to ask your questions. You need to make sure you end up with a doctor with whom you are comfortable!

Two final notes to this introduction (if you will pardon the double oxymoron):

#1. Most books dealing with vitamins and other nutrient supplements are either encyclopedic in nature, covering every possible vitamin, mineral or herb for every disease known to man or beast,[10] or they are promoting a specific supplement such as MSM or SAMe, or they are concerned with general matters such as aging or skin health or falling hair. It seems to me some good purpose is to be served in taking on a specific malady such as peripheral neuropathy, keeping it in fairly narrow focus, and wringing dry all the nutrient information that can be

---

[10] Curiously, peripheral neuropathy is usually omitted. Maybe no one else believes it's real. We know better.

found on the one topic. If you are a fellow PNer I hope you will gain from my having attempted to do so.

#2. As in my other two books I have used many content footnotes. There was much material I came across that I wanted to share with you which, though important, was often somewhat tangential to the matter then being discussed. I thought on balance this approach should be less distracting to you than always sticking ideas in the middle of the text which would be somewhat off the point and which might break your thought train. The editors at the *Chicago Manual of Style*—the supposed "final word" on such matters—think it is not very good form to use many content footnotes. I figure, though, when it's your own book you can break a few rules if you want to. However, as I wrote in *Toes and Woes*, if these footnotes all seem a little overwhelming, just keep your eyes focused above the horizontal lines at the bottom of the pages— unless your curiosity gets the better of you.

Chapter 1

The Uses of Supplements

Our bodies need certain vitamins and other nutrients in minimum amounts to maintain adequate health. These so-called **essential nutrients** are substances that we cannot make ourselves and that we need to function properly. They all must come from food or from dietary supplements.

The essential nutrients include 23 minerals, 12 vitamins, 8 amino acids, and 2 fatty acids. From these, a healthy body makes other substances required for functioning. Individuals may derive additional benefits from a diet that includes non-essential nutrients.

Deficiency of any essential nutrient results in alteration of normal cell, tissue, and body function, accompanied by symptoms of deteriorating health. Deficiency of each particular essential nutrient has its own set of symptoms. Prolonged deficiencies can possibly lead, through progressive deterioration, to death.

Various guidelines have been used to determine the levels of vitamins and minerals that are supposedly sufficient for "normal functioning." However, determining proper daily intake is not an exact science. Standards set by governments around the world often differ.

In the United States a set of standards has been adopted called **Reference Daily Intakes**, or **RDIs**. They are meant to represent "adequate essential nutrition" for adults and children four or more years old (a range, incidentally, that could put the nutritional needs of a 50 pound child in the same category as a 150 pound adult). RDIs are used in calculating the "% Daily Values" which must appear on supplement labels.

The typical American diet does not supply these nutrients in the amounts indicated by the RDIs. In the early 1990s a number of studies were requested by Congress to gather information on the use and need of "dietary supplements."[1] The findings were rather astounding. Of the thousands of people studied, hardly any were getting from their diets the full Recommended Daily Allowances (the predecessor of RDIs) of ten key vitamins and minerals identified by science as essential to health.

The nutritional shortfalls from typical or average diets are about as true today as ten years ago. Researchers at

---

[1] "Dietary supplement" is a term used in federal regulations to mean a product that is intended to supplement the diet and which constitutes or contains one or more of the following: a vitamin, a mineral, an herb or other botanical, an amino acid, a metabolite, a concentrate, an extract, a constituent, any other dietary substance for use by humans to supplement the diet by increasing the total dietary intake, or any combination of the foregoing. Like many others I prefer to use the term "nutrient supplement" which means much the same thing but better emphasizes the reason for taking one of these substances in the first place.

the University of California, Berkeley, recently reported that only 9% of people eat the five daily servings of fruit and vegetables recommended by experts.

There are various reasons for this: most of us are too busy to pay proper attention to always eating well-balanced meals; foods are over-processed in their preparation and preservation; valuable minerals have often been leached from soils in which food is grown; harmful nutrient-destroying chemicals are frequently added to these soils or sprayed directly on plants to increase production (a few years ago researchers at the U.S. Department of Agriculture found that conventional nitrogen fertilizer reduced vitamin C levels in some food crops by as much as one third), etc., etc.

General Nutrient Supplementation

Even if we were more careful as to what we eat and even if all of the foods we consume retained all the nutrients nature intended to be there and even if all the RDIs were fully met, the nutrients we take in would still not be enough for many of us. (As an example, a boiled egg supplies .7 micrograms of vitamin B12; it is widely believed that *1000* micrograms should be taken daily for peripheral neuropathy.) Genetic factors, age, environmental conditions, stress, smoking and drinking habits, existing deficiencies, exercise requirements, disease prevention, or just the wish to be extra fit, all make **nutrient supple-**

mentation necessary or desirable.[2] (As an added plus and motivator, supplements provide measurable amounts of nutrients and are often calorie and fat-free.)

For these reasons, and maybe even more importantly because many do not believe that even a well-balanced diet delivers enough nutrients and/or that in any event the RDIs are high enough to be good guides, a multi-billion dollar supplement industry has developed in the United States. This industry offers hundreds of supplements and thousands of combinations in the form of pills or tablets, capsules, softgels, lozenges, liquids, powders, and "nutrition bars."

A report prepared in October 2000 by the Hankin investment banking firm said that the supplement industry grew at a 15% compounded rate through most of the 90's. They expect the trend to continue, observing "the public awareness of the positive effects of vitamins and nutritional supplements on health has been heightened by widely publicized reports of scientific findings supporting such [health] claims." One purveyor of nutritional products claims, in fact, that nearly 50% of Americans

---

[2] Many years ago Roger Williams, Ph.D., developed the concept of "biochemical individuality" in pointing out that people are highly *individualistic* in the amounts of nutrients they need.

A study, "Is There a Metabolic Basis for Dietary Supplementation?," cites a couple of examples of special *group* requirements: elderly people have a greater need for vitamin D and B12; pregnant women have a greater need of folate to help prevent neural tube defects in their babies (abnormal embryonic developments producing congenital malformations); and athletes who exercise intensively sometimes require more antioxidant supplements than most to overcome reactive oxygen derivatives. *American Journal of Nutrition* (2000 Aug; 72 (2 Suppl): 507S-11S).

use vitamin supplements every day. (A dash of cold water was thrown on all this exuberance by a report in *Nutrition Business Journal*, which said herbal sales had grown by just 1% in 2000 after enjoying annual gains in the "12–17% range" for a number of years.)

Therapeutic Nutrient Supplementation

The market just described is largely for supplements used for general nutritional uses. The market for nutrients used specifically for **therapeutic purposes**—that is for the **treatment** of **disease states**—is surely just a small fraction of the broader nutritional market.

Typically much higher nutrient doses are required for treatment than when taken for general health purposes. To give one example: the RDI of vitamin E is 30 IUs (international units) daily. When used as an antioxidant supplement for therapeutic purposes, as indicated later in this book, the typical recommended dosage is *400 to 800* IU daily.

Knowledgeable professionals believe that the market for supplements used therapeutically will increase faster than the overall supplement market. This is because the body of scientific evidence concerning the efficacy of **nutrient treatments,** which for economic reasons as previously noted has been developed mainly outside of this country, is becoming more widely known and accepted here.

Nutrient supplementation is often used in neuropathy treatment where there is an **existing deficiency** of a needed nutrient in a particular individual. (To use yet another term, medical professionals sometimes refer to this as "substitutive" or "replacement therapy.") A few of the clinical studies reported here and in *Toes and Soles* and *Toes and Woes* deal with instances where nutrients were administered specifically for that purpose. Where a deficiency *is* determined to be a cause, primary or secondary, aggressive treatment with supplementation is usually indicated.[3]

But often there is no specific cause for the neuropathy identified in clinical studies. In fact in many of the investigations discussed in *Toes and Soles* and *Toes and Woes* and later in this book where nutrients were therapeutically used with success, the investigators *did not even consider* whether there was a pre-existing deficiency of the nutrient being administered, at least according to the study reports. If in fact the existence of a deficiency was the driving premise in these studies, it was curiously unstated! Is it possible that in all of these studies, some of which were otherwise quite carefully designed, that the critical factor of pre-existing deficiency had been overlooked? Clearly not, I think.

There are some in the medical community who will

---

[3] It should also be noted that even though there might not be an actual deficiency of the nutrient in the body, something else important may be in short supply that is restored with supplementation, or the nutrient performs some other specific, identifiable function. See, e.g., a study performed at the Russian Medical Academy, Moscow, where the administration of alpha-lipoic acid (ALA) was found to have normalized a nitric oxide metabolite, thereby producing a positive effect for patients with PN. *Bulletin of Experimental Biology and Medicine* (2000 Oct: 130 (10): 986–90).

still argue that there is no point in using nutrient supplements unless there is actual proof that the deficiency of a needed nutrient caused the neuropathy. (Such arguments tend to reflect the same mindset as the director of one of the country's leading diabetes centers when he said that if a specific deficiency can't be found, "the vitamins will just go down the drain in your urine."[4]) Also, that kind of thinking ignores the many instances where a particular nutrient, of which there is no known or proven deficiency, may foster or enhance the action of another nutrient, or in some other manner initiate or catalyze a metabolic process which produces a beneficial result.

One has to wonder whether these nutrient minimalists would have us believe that all of us **idiopaths**, whose neuropathy causations are by definition unknown, were **idiotic** in taking nutrients, and that if the supplements happened to work, well, we were just lucky in matching a particular nutrient to a particular deficiency.[5] Presumably they would then suggest that our "idiopathicness" was due to faulty testing all along.

Moreover, this fixation on **deficiency** as a *sine qua non*

---

[4] "Neuropathy Nerve Damage-An Update," Joslin Diabetes Center, 1999. There is some truth in the remark but not quite in the way it was intended. The fact is that our bodies don't use everything we eat to best advantage. (That's why going to the bathroom is a normal function.) But ingesting supplements does beneficially increase blood levels, and sometimes tissue levels, of those nutrients for subsequent use even though the process isn't 100% efficient.

[5] Maybe those who say nutrients only help with PN where there was a deficiency should also say that if Neurontin or Elavil are providing pain relief there must have been a deficiency of Neurontin or Elavil in our bodies! (Okay, okay, I know the analogy is a little specious but it sounded so good I had to include it.)

for the use of nutrients would make somewhat pointless the administration of substances such as alpha-lipoic acid and acetyl-l-carnitine (both discussed later). These nutrients have sometimes proven extremely helpful in dealing with PN but, not being vital to bodily functions in the same sense as are many of the vitamins and minerals, do not have established requirements that might result in recognized deficiencies. (Incidentally, Richard N. Podell, M.D., who has studied alpha-lipoic acid extensively, claims a study discussed later in this book "provides the first clear evidence that nutritional treatment alone can reverse the course of autonomic neuropathy"!)

Anyway, not all clinicians accept the argument that you have to have a pre-existing deficiency for nutrient supplementation to work. Japanese investigators have found, for example, that even though vitamin B6 deficiency *had specifically not* been established in cases they had under review, supplementation of B6 was nevertheless effective in improving "PN symptoms of *various aetiologies* [emphasis added]." [6]

I came across another interesting study which, if believed, would seem to make the issue of nutrient deficiencies as causal factors for neuropathy almost irrelevant in

---

[6] *Nephrology, Dialysis, Transplantation* (2000 Sep; 15 (9): 1410–13).

Jerry R. Mendell, M.D., in his excellent chapter entitled "Vitamin Deficiencies: Cobalamin (Vitamin B12), Vitamin E (Tocopherol), and Thiamine (Vitamin B1)", appearing in *Diagnosis and Management of Peripheral Nerve Disorders* (Mendell, Kissel and Cornblath, 2001 Oxford University Press), claimed, in fact, that "vitamin deficiency is a relatively uncommon cause of peripheral neuropathy but may occur in relation to deficiency of cobalamin, vitamin E, and possibly thiamine." (p. 545).

any event. German investigators tested the levels of vitamins A, E, beta carotene, B1, B2, B6, B12, and folate, in 29 elderly women with Type 2 diabetes. Seventeen of them had diabetic neuropathy and 12 did not. The investigators determined that the vitamin levels did not vary between the two groups and concluded there was a lack of association between pre-existing vitamin levels and diabetic neuropathy. The investigators did not take the next, what might have seemed logical, step of giving nutrients to the ladies who had neuropathies—perhaps not surprising since based on their testing they might well have thought it would be pointless.[7]

There is a lesson to be learned from the animal kingdom here also. There are many clinical studies concerning neuropathies induced in otherwise perfectly healthy laboratory rats where nutrients were then administered by the investigators immediately after the induction. Obvi-

---

[7] *Medizinische Klinik* (1993 Aug 15: 88(8): 453–57).

Many studies covered in this book concern "diabetic neuropathy." The question arises as to the applicability of conclusions drawn from these studies to other neuropathies. I made the point in *Toes and Woes* that, in so far as pain (and probably other symptomatic) treatments are concerned, there should be a great deal of correlation since the nerve or myelin damage which created the pain or other problem is the same, regardless of the cause. However, where there are special circumstances, such as the deficiency of a particular nutrient contributing to glucose intolerance (see, e.g., the discussion later on chromium), leading to the "diabetic neuropathy," or where there is some other problem peculiar to diabetics (for example, the difficulty that those with diabetes have in converting linoleic acid to GLA, thereby creating a greater need for GLA supplementation), the applicability of study conclusions may be more limited. I suspect, however, that *most* nutrient treatments that work for diabetic neuropathies will be beneficial for other kinds. Certainly it would be helpful, however, if a few studies could be directed specifically at this question.

ously there were no pre-existing vitamin deficiencies causing the neuropathies because the little fellows had been
getting along just fine before they were traumatized.
Where good treatment results were obtained from the administration of nutrients, as they were in many of these
studies, you would have to attribute it to something other
than correcting a deficiency.

As an aside, I think there's an irony that some medical
professionals won't consider using supplements for treating peripheral neuropathy at the same time they know
they are being used successfully for more serious ailments
such as cancer or heart disease.[8] The paradox is that for
these more serious disease states there *are* conventional
medical therapies that can actually help overcome the
condition, yet doctors are still using nutrient supplementations for curative purposes. For peripheral neuropathy,
where there are *no* medical therapies that can hope to
cure, it seems to me that there should be a particular interest on the part of doctors in trying supplements that
just might restore their patients' health.[9]

---

[8] There are clinical studies that clearly recognize the use of nutrient
supplements, at least as adjunctive treatments, for these diseases.
See, e.g., "Tumor Cell Growth Inhibition," reporting on the use of vitamin K to inhibit the growth of cancer cells (*Journal of Molecular
Biology*, 2001 Dec; 314 (4): 765–72), and "Nutritional Strategies in
Cardiovascular Disease Control: An Update on Vitamins and Condi-
tionally Essential Nutrients," reporting on the use of vitamins E, C,
B6, folate, and CoQ10, as beneficial adjunctive strategies in control-
ling cardiovascular disease. *Progress in Cardiovascular Nursing*
(1999 Autumn; 14 (4): 124–29).

[9] In a provocative article, "Nutritional Therapy at the Crossroads,"
Jack Challem, who was mentioned in a previous footnote, wrote:

"We have reached a time when the scientific evidence supporting the
preventive and therapeutic use of vitamins, minerals, and other food

The reason I am dwelling on all of this is hopefully to dispel this idea put out by some that there is, at best, only a narrow role for supplements. I think it's a shame for people not to take advantage of a strategy that might really be beneficial when they are told, after batteries of tests, that no specific nutrient deficiency was found which warrants nutrient administration. ("Here's your prescription, Madam, for three months more of methadone to help with all the pain that won't let you sleep. I'm sorry there is nothing further medicine can do for you—you looked all right in all of our tests.")

Let me make a point here. I'm not arguing against medications for peripheral neuropathy where necessary and where they can help. I still need Neurontin, for example; happily I just don't always need as much as I used to (often 600 mg daily rather than always 900 mg previously), based largely, I am convinced, on the benefits from the supplements I'm taking. Also, my neuropathy does not cause *anywhere* near the pain I used to have.

The existing mindset on the part of some against nutrient supplements is not unreasonable, in a way. It has doubtlessly, and unfortunately, been brought on by the nutrient supplement industry itself. There has been much too much hype used in the past to promote products. Even now this is a problem in spite of the fact that there are stringent federal rules concerning claims that can properly be made for nutritional supplements. (Our mailbox at home is often stuffed with colorful, multi-page brochures

---

factors is literally overwhelming. It's all in the medical literature." (*Journal of Orthomolecular Medicine*, 1994 9(3): 145–50).

trumpeting "miracle cures" from herbal and other combinations, guaranteed to change our lives.)

Recent events such as the establishment of a federal Office of Dietary Supplements at the National Institutes of Health will help inject a little professionalism in this regard, though, and eliminate some of the fluff. The Office's mission as stated is "to strengthen knowledge and understanding of dietary supplements by evaluating scientific information, stimulating and supporting research, disseminating research results, and educating the public to foster an enhanced quality of life and health for the U.S. population." ODS has a data base that at the time this was written contained over 639,000 scientific citations and abstracts concerning dietary supplements.

Please keep in mind, by the way, that this book is about *supplements*, substances meant to *supplement* the nutrients we obtain naturally from what we eat. We should start by stressing foods in our diets that offer the highest values of the nutrients we need in order that our immune systems are strengthened. (Still it might be noted that supplement forms of nutrients often yield **higher efficiencies** of **digestion** and **absorption** than when nutrients are bound in foods.[10])

In the discussions of the various nutrients in this book general information is provided as to preferred food sources. There are books full of very *detailed* information

---

[10] See Ball, G.F.M. 1998. *Bioavailability and Analysis of Vitamins in Foods*. (London: Chapman & Hall, 26). Also see the discussion of bioavailability in Chapter 5.

in this regard. One particularly helpful one is the *Nutrition Almanac*.[11] It offers a "Table of Food Composition" which sets out a complete nutritional analysis of over 1600 foods, indicating the amounts in these foods of the vitamins, minerals, and other nutrients discussed in this book.

Following the last chapter are four nutrient tables reprinted with the permission of the Council for Responsible Nutrition (a trade association representing more than 100 companies in the dietary supplement industry). The first two compare the current RDIs with new DRIs and Uls (you gotta love all these acronyms) for vitamins and minerals. DRIs stand for Dietary Reference Intakes. These are dietary recommendations said to be the possible basis for updating the RDIs. Uls are the upper limits considered to be safe.

The next two tables provide historical comparisons for vitamin and mineral RDIs, RDAs, and DRIs, from 1968 through 2001. In general it may be observed that the recommendations for vitamins C, D, and K have increased over this period while those for vitamin A, the B vitamins and their cousins, and vitamin E, have gone down. You will note about as many recommendations for minerals have decreased as have increased over this time span.

---

[11] Kirschman 1996. Mc Graw Hill, 4th Ed.

Chapter 2

Vitamins

Vitamins are **organic nutrients** vital for proper growth and maintenance of health. Unlike carbohydrates, fats, and proteins, they are not sources of energy. Instead they function as **enzymes** or **catalysts** or **co-factors** in chemical reactions which continually take place in our bodies, including cell production, tissue repair, and other vital metabolic processes.

Vitamins are classified as being either **fat-soluble** or **water-soluble.** Vitamins A, D, E, and K are examples of the former. They remain in body tissues for a relatively long period of time after being ingested and are absorbed by the body using processes that closely parallel the absorption of fat. Water-soluble vitamins (exemplified by vitamins B and C) are retained for only short periods before being flushed out. Consequently, they need to be frequently replenished. Because they are readily excreted, toxicity risks are lessened.

The only three vitamins that can be **manufactured** in the body are D, K, and the vitamin B cousin, biotin. The rest must be supplied by food or supplements.

The emphasis in this chapter is on those vitamins for which there is **credible scientific evidence** that supplementation will or might provide **neuropathic benefits**. Consequently vitamins A and D, which are both important nutritionally but which do not play particularly important roles for PNers, are not dealt with here.[1] (Of course you may still need to supplement your regular diet with these nutrients for other health reasons.)

Incidentally, where RDIs or dosages are mentioned in the following discussions, it is critical to pay attention to whether the indicated level is for "mcg," "mg," or "g," and to differentiate accordingly. Mcgs, the smallest units, are micrograms. One thousand mcgs equal one mg or one milligram. One thousand milligrams equal in turn one g or one gram. Capisce?

The B Complex

The group referred to as the **B complex** is a set of 12 somewhat related substances which because of their water-solubility, as mentioned before, must be regularly replenished.

Together, the B vitamins have a broad range of functions. These include maintenance of **myelin**, which is the

---

[1] I came across a French study which suggested that vitamin A, together with vitamin E, was essential in preventing patients from developing secondary effects such as neuropathy following treatment for a rare genetic disease. *Annales d'endocrinologie* (2000 May; 61(2): 125–29).There is also an English study acknowledging that retinoic acid, a metabolite (i.e., a substance produced by a metabolic process) of vitamin A, is important in the control of axon outgrowth. *Proceedings of the National Academy of Science U S A* (1991 May 1; 88(9): 3666–70).

covering around nerve fibers. A breakdown of myelin can cause a large and devastating variety of neurological symptoms such as peripheral neuropathy. (*Toes and Soles* and *Toes and Woes* discuss in detail nerve cells and fibers, myelin disorders, and injuries that result in neuropathy.) B vitamins are also key to helping in the production of energy from other nutrients we ingest. Three members of this group, namely folic acid, pyridoxine (B6), and cobalamin (B12), work together to keep homocysteine levels low. This is quite important since high homocysteine levels are associated with heart disease.

Some B vitamins prevent certain birth problems (such as neural tube defects as previously mentioned), maintain healthy red blood cells, support immune function, regulate cell growth, aid in the production of hormones, and may have a role in preventing some types of cancer. They also function in the maintenance of healthy skin, hair, and nails.

A few of the B vitamins have unique functions that allow a particular deficiency to be readily identified. Usually, however, they **work together** so well that it may be difficult to determine which ones are in short-supply in a given case.[2]

---

[2] Sometimes testing combinations will reveal which one is working particularly well. A 1996 study considered the effect of vitamin B complex supplementation on neurotransmission and neurite outgrowth (the latter being the ability of neuronal axons to grow towards other neurons following injury). The investigators found that the combination of three of the B vitamins (B1, B6 and B12) had a more salutary effect than just two of them (B1 and B12), giving a thumbs-up to the combination using B6. *General Pharmacology* (1996 Sep; 27 (6): 995-1000).

In general, low B vitamin levels will cause profound fatigue and an assortment of **neurologic manifestations** which may include weakness, poor balance, confusion, irritability, memory loss, nervousness, tingling of the limbs, and loss of coordination. Depression may be an early sign of significantly low levels of pyridoxine (B6) and possibly other B vitamins. Additional symptoms of vitamin B deficiency are sleep disturbances, nausea, poor appetite, frequent infections, and skin lesions.[3]

A strong **synergistic** effect is produced when vitamins in the B complex are used in combination. In one study supporting this idea, various therapeutic combinations of vitamins B2, B6, and B12 were considered. An investigation involving 234 doctors in private practices treating 1,149 patients with polyneuropathy, neuralgia, radiculopathy (a pathological condition of the nerve roots), neuritis associated with pain, and *paresthesias* (numb or prickling sensations) was undertaken. The end points evaluated were intensity of pain, muscle weakness affecting legs, and *paresthesia*. The investigators found clear symptomatic improvement from the use of these combinations. At a second examination approximately three weeks after initiation of treatments, a positive effect on pain in particular was observed in 69% of the cases. Similar observations were made for *paresthesias* and muscular weakness in the legs.[4]

---

[3] Much of the information in this and the three preceding paragraphs was based on material in the *Gale Encyclopedia of Alternative Medicine* (Krapp et al. December 2000).

[4] *Fortschritte der Medizin* (1992 Oct 20; 110 (29): 544–48). See also the study reported in *General Pharmacology* above.

In another study investigators found that several patients with peripheral neuropathies resulting from **surgeries** had benefited from "vitamin B complex replacement."[5]

Dr. Ward Dean, author of the book, *Smart Drugs and Nutrients,*[6] mentions a 1996 double-blind study of 24 diabetic patients who suffered from PN in which a high-dose B complex regimen was used: thiamin, 320 mg/d for the first 2 weeks, and 120 mg/d thereafter; vitamin B6, 720 mg/d for the first 2 weeks, and 270 mg/d thereafter; and vitamin B12, 2,000 mcg/d for the first 2 weeks and then 750 mcg/d thereafter. According to the principal investigator the treatment resulted in significant improvement in nerve conduction velocity in the peroneal nerve (a small nerve associated with the fibula and innervating certain muscle and skin areas of the leg and foot) and an improvement of the "vibration perception threshold."[7]

Although B vitamins should be taken in combination (such as to be found in a typical B 50 or B 100 formulation),

---

[5] *The American Journal of Gastroenterology* (1983 Jun; 78 (6): 321–23).

[6] *Smart Publications,* August 1991.

[7] Results from clinical studies tend to be directed to and stated in terms of effects of a particular therapy on subjective symptoms such as *paresthesia* and pain, or on objective parameters such as vibration threshold and nerve conduction velocity, and oftentimes on both subjective and objective "outcomes." Nerve conduction velocity, or NCV, incidentally is a measure of how fast electrical impulses flow through a nerve. It is related to the diameter of the nerve and, sometimes, to the degree of its myelination (the presence of a myelin sheath on the axon).

a couple of them are so important that consideration ought to be given to additional amounts for a PNer's regime. Also when a more **bioavailable** form (i.e., more readily available to the particular body tissues where needed) is to be had which offers special benefits, it might be desirable to add that nutrient form separately. This is all discussed below.

1. B1

Also known as **thiamin** (sometimes spelled thiamine), vitamin B1 was the first vitamin to be discovered, thus its B1 designation. In the late 19th century scientists observed that animals fed a diet of polished rice developed beriberi and that putting rice husks back in their feed could cure the disease. Pure thiamin was isolated for the first time in 1926. In 1934 the actual structure of the substance was discovered with the first synthesis occurring in 1936.

As with other water-soluble vitamins, B1 in the common forms (thiamin hydrochloride or thiamin mononitrate) is not stored in the body to any great extent and must be **obtained daily** from food or other sources. (Thirty milligrams (mg) are stored in body tissue. Laurence Kinsella, M.D., a noted authority on nutrition and neuropathy who wrote the Foreword for this book, says that thiamin can be depleted from the body in as little as 3 weeks.)

After it is ingested the vitamin is carried by the **circulatory system** to the liver, kidneys, and heart. It may then combine with manganese resulting in an active enzyme that breaks down complex carbohydrates into simple sugars. Incidentally, alcohol easily destroys B1. (Dr. Kinsella, just referred to, has written extensively on the associations between alcohol, thiamin, and neuropathy.) Smoking depletes the vitamin as well.

A deficiency can cause either "wet beriberi," in which congestive heart failure is the primary symptom, or "dry beriberi," in which peripheral neuropathy is the primary symptom, depending on the percentage of carbohydrates in the diet. (Deficiencies preferentially affect the nervous and cardiac tissues because thiamin is bound less strongly there, with the possibility of myelin sheath degeneration and axon impairment producing the peripheral neuropathy.) The vagal nerve, which enervates the gastrointestinal tract, heart and larynx, is particularly affected.

Thiamin is used principally in the **conversion** of amino acids, fats, and carbohydrates into **energy**. It is also vital for normal development of skin and hair, blood production, and immune functions. The key importance of vitamin B1 for us is its ability to synthesize an important neurotransmitter—**acetylcholine**—in the nervous system that allows nerve impulses to travel from one nerve cell to another.[8] Thiamin also has a role in maintaining nerve cell membranes. There are several clinical and anecdotal reports concerning its usefulness for dealing with peripheral neuropathy in this regard.[9]

---

[8] "The neurotrophic function of thiamin may be due to its coenzymatic role in a biochemical reaction and/or its specific function on neurotransmission and nerve conduction." *Japanese Journal of Pharmacology* (1995 Jul; 68 (3): 349–52).

[9] It has long been recognized, of course, that a thiamin deficiency can cause peripheral neuropathy. See, e.g., *European Archives of Psychiatry and Neurological Sciences* (1985; 234 (6): 390–94).

In a study performed at the University of Dar es Salaam, Tanzania, the clinical response to therapeutic doses of thiamin and pyridoxine (vitamin B6) was determined in 200 diabetic patients with peripheral neuropathy. They were randomly separated into two groups. One hundred (group A) were given treatment with both thiamin (25 mg/day) and pyridoxine (50 mg/day). The second hundred (group B) were given an identical tablet containing just 1 mg/day each of thiamin and pyridoxine. Pain, numbness, *paresthesia,* and impairment of lower extremity sensation were all tracked. Four weeks after starting treatment the severity of peripheral neuropathy symptoms decreased in 48.9% of patients in group A compared with 11.4% in group B, indicating that the larger doses produced significantly greater benefits.[10]

The foregoing study did not indicate in which form the thiamin was taken but presumably it was in one of the more common—either thiamin hydrochloride or thiamin mononitrate. The well-known Atkins Institute for Complementary Medicine similarly failed to make a distinction when reporting a 50% benefit rate for their patients suffering from diabetic neuropathy following thiamin administration.[11]

There are lipid-soluble forms of thiamin which are superior to water-soluble thiamin hydrochloride or thiamin

---

[10] *East Africa Medical Journal* (1997 Dec; 74(12): 803–808).

[11] They also referred to a 12-week German study where apparently plain vanilla B1—together with other B vitamins—was given in high dosages—320 mg daily—to patients with diabetic neuropathy with successful outcomes. V. Frydl et al *Medwelt* (1989; 40: 1484–86).

mononitrate because of the **greater bioavailability** of
the lipid-soluble forms; a larger portion of the active ingredient in those forms is going to be absorbed and metabolized in tissues where needed rather than uselessly
excreted. Accordingly, the thiamin in the fat-soluble
forms should be more beneficial in dealing with peripheral neuropathy.

Most of the lipid-soluble thiamin studies concern a
substance called **benfotiamine.** Several were reported
in *Toes and Woes*, and two additional ones are mentioned
here.

The classic and much cited investigation on the particular benefits of benfotiamine for treating neuropathy was
performed by H. Stracke et al.[12] In a double-blind, randomized, controlled study, benfotiamine, together with
B6/B12, was administered over a period of 12 weeks to 24
patients with diabetic neuropathy. The researchers found
a significant improvement in nerve conduction velocity
and improvement in "vibration perception."

The Stracke study was followed in 1997 by one in Bul-
garia which compared the therapeutic efficacy of "Milgamma" tablets (50 mg benfotiamine and .25 mg [sic] vitamin B12) with conventional vitamin B complex tablets.
Forty-five diabetes patients with peripheral neuropathy
were divided into two groups and received the different
treatments over a three-month period. At the end of the
study the investigators said that "statistically significant
relief of both background and peak neuropathic pain was

---

[12] *Experimental and Clinical Endocrinology and Diabetes* (1996; 104
(4): 311–16).

achieved in all of the Milgamma-treated patients and vibration perception thresholds dramatically improved," while "symptom improvement was insignificant" among those on the conventional B complex regimen. The investigators proclaimed the Milgamma tablets "an indispensable element in the therapeutic regimen of patients with painful diabetic neuropathy."[13]

Other studies performed in Russia, Germany, and Hungary as reported in *Toes and Woes* reached substantially the same conclusion.[14] More recent investigations affirmed the superior efficacy of benfotiamine over other thiamin forms, one in which benfotiamine was tested against thiamin nitrate in a randomized study of 20 end-stage renal disease patients[15] and the other involving a study of three groups of broiler chickens given three different thiamin forms (guess which chickens turned out to be the plumpest).[16]

A similar conclusion was reached in the United States where the **bioequivalence** (i.e., the degree to which the same bioavailability and physiological effects are provided) of three fat-soluble thiamin preparations—benfo-

---

[13] *Folia Medica* (1997; 39 (4): 5–10).

[14] See *Zh Nevrol Psikhiatr Im S S Korsakova* (1998; 98(9): 30–32) (an "amelioration of the neuropathic condition" in 93% of the cases); *Alcohol and Alcoholism* (1998 Nov-Dec; 33 (6): 631–38) ("Benfotiamine led to a significant improvement in alcoholic polyneuropathy"); *Arzneimittelforschung* (1999 Mar; 49(3): 220–24) ("those patients receiving the highest doses of benfotiamine at three different dose levels, received the greatest benefit").

[15] *European Journal of Clinical Pharmacology* (2000 Jun; 56 (3): 251–57).

[16] *International Journal for Vitamin and Nutrition Research* (2000 Dec; 70 (6): 311–16).

tiamine and two others—were compared using seven volunteers with polyneuropathies. The researchers said that, "From our results it can be concluded that oral administration of benfotiamine is best suitable for therapeutical purposes owing to its excellent absorption characteristics." (A significant feature of the test, in my opinion, was that the investigators were studying these three thiamin derivatives as **neurotropic agents**—i.e., assessing their possible capability to promote **nerve regeneration**, not just for pain or other symptomatic relief).[17]

This last study is particularly interesting because one of the preparations which benfotiamine was tested against is a substance with the technical name "thiamin tetrahydrofurfuryl disulfide." (Trying saying that fast a couple of times! In fact, try saying it just once.) Even though it did not test as well as benfotiamine, TTFD (a.k.a. **allithiamine**), which naturally occurs in the allium species of plants, has been found superior to the usual water-soluble forms of thiamin. In fact an early study performed in Japan concluded that the oral administration of allithiamine compared very favorably with the **parenteral** (intravenous or subcutaneous injection) administration of water-soluble thiamins.[18]

Alan R. Gaby, M.D., and Trina M. Seligman, N.D., re-

---

[17] *International Journal of Clinical Pharmacology and Therapeutics* (1998 Apr; 36(4): 216–21). An earlier study assessing the bioequivalence of benfotiamine compared with thiamin mononitrate found "significantly improved bioavailability" from the former when given to 10 healthy young men at a dosage of only 40% of the latter. *Annals of Nutrition & Metabolism* (1991; 35(5): 292–96).

[18] *Journal of Nutritional Science and Vitaminology* (1976 Aug; 22 SUPPL: 63–68).

ported in a 1996 paper on "The Treatment of Diabetes with Natural Therapeutics," a study of 24 patients who had received daily either a placebo or 320 mg of allithiamine, plus 720 mg of pyridoxine and 2.0 mg of vitamin B12. After two weeks, the dosages of the vitamins were reduced by about two-thirds. After 12 weeks of treatment, there was said to have been a significant improvement in nerve-conduction velocity in the vitamin-treated group compared with the placebo group. No significant side effects were seen.[19]

Dr. Lark Lands, a noted nutrition expert, has also made supportive comments concerning the use of allithiamine in managing neuropathy in HIV-positive people.

The point of bringing allithiamine into the picture, even if according to one study the other fat-soluble form of thiamin, benfotiamine, may be superior, is simply that it is not *possible* to buy the benfotiamine in the U.S. If you insist on that particular fat-soluble formulation, you will have to order it from East Europe. Allithiamine, however, is available from at least a few suppliers here. One is Ecological Formulas and they were selling a bottle of 60 capsules of 50 mg for $16.95 at the time this was written (1-800-289-8487). Gaines Nutrition was selling their formulation of allithiamine in the same amounts and strength for $15.95 (1-800-830-7139). The Vitamin

---

[19] Published in 1996 by Project Cure in association with Bastyr University's National Public Medicine Program. (Bastyr is a natural health sciences institution in Kenmore, Washington.)

The author of the Foreword to this book, Laurence J. Kinsella, M.D., points out that 720 mg of pyridoxine or B6 is a dangerously high amount.

Shoppe was advertising allithiamine at $12.76 for 60 cap-
sules. (There may be more places to buy this but not every
supplier handles allithiamine.)

Although the current RDI for thiamin is 20 mg daily
(which would be based on the common forms), the dosage
recommended by suppliers of allithiamine for **general
nutritional purposes** is one or two 50 mg capsules
daily. For **therapeutic purposes**, however, a daily intake of 200–300 mg of allithiamine would not seem too
much based on the clinical studies cited above. The common water soluble forms of vitamin B1 have actually
been used in therapeutic doses of up to a gram a day.

Vitamin B1 is considered quite safe and I did not find
any adverse drug interactions reported. As always,
though, it is advisable to consult a medical professional
prior to using this vitamin in supplemental form for
therapeutic purposes.

Incidentally, good natural food sources of B1 include
yeast, peanuts, peas, beans, and seeds. (The allithiamine
form occurs naturally in garlic but you will lose friends if
you try to take your full quota that way; garlic oil capsules are an odorless option, however.) The milling of cereals removes most of the thiamin so white flour and
breakfast cereals are usually enriched with the vitamin.
Some foods are said to **impair** its absorption, including
fish, shrimp, clams, mussels, and the herb, horsetail.

2. B2

This vitamin, also known as **riboflavin**, is important in
the production of **body energy**. The special significance

of **B2** to us, though, lies in its ability to both help with the conversion of B6 to a form we can use, and help generate **glutathione**. The latter is an enzyme that acts as one of our most significant antioxidants. (This enzyme is a carefully designed molecule of protein that can "quench" free radicals[20] but needs both vitamin E, the mineral selenium, and other factors in order to do its work.)

A deficiency of riboflavin can result in **nerve disorders** and a **degeneration of myelin sheaths**. It works closely with folic acid, pantothenic acid (B5) and vitamin B12. It can also lessen the symptoms of pantothenic acid and zinc deficiencies.

A "neuropathy epidemic" occurred in Cuba in 1991 in which 51,000 cases of PN were reported. Afterwards a survey was conducted in a random sample of smokers and non-smokers living in Havana. The aim was to investigate "metabolic and dietary parameters" in the two groups of volunteers that could explain the underlying mechanisms. The investigators concluded "low biologically avail-

---

[20] Free radicals are highly reactive oxygen fragments or damaged molecules lacking one or more electrons. They are created in the body by normal chemical processes such as the conversion of food into energy. Free radicals can also be produced in dangerous amounts by irritants such as cigarette smoke, pesticides, air pollution, ultraviolet light and radiation, as well as by stress and over exercising. Because the free-radical molecule "wants" its full complement of electrons, it reacts with any molecule from which it can take an electron. These give-away molecules are found in certain key components such as fat, protein or DNA. By swiping these electrons, free radicals damage the associated cells and cause oxidative stress. According to some experts, this not infrequently leads to peripheral neuropathy and other disorders. Antioxidants neutralize the free radicals by giving up their electrons easily and restoring the natural balance.

able quantities of carotenoids [these are nutrients occurring in red or orange plants—such as carrots—and
convertible into vitamin A] and **riboflavin** from low dietary intakes and depletion through smoking [were] the
main precipitating factors" of the huge number of neuropathy cases.[21]

Natural food sources include organ meats, yeast, eggs,
nuts, and green leafy vegetables. The current RDI for B1
is 1.7 mg. For therapeutic purposes, dosages as high as
400 mg daily have been used.

Riboflavin is quite safe and has not been found toxic at
levels as high as 1000 mg daily. The only reported drug
interaction I found was with oral contraceptives (I don't
use them); in that case it is said you may need additional
amounts of B2.

3. B3

Vitamin B3 or **niacin** (a.k.a. **nicotinic acid**) is often
used to reduce high cholesterol levels and treat high blood
pressure, acne, and alcoholism.[22] It is also recommended
for weight reduction since it helps stabilize blood sugar

---

[21] *International Journal for Vitamin and Nutrition Research* (2000
May; 70(3): 126–38). Dr. Laurence Kinsella, in commenting to me
about this study, said it was likely there was a polynutritional
deficiency in Cuba at that time, similar to an epidemic in Jamaica in
the 1880s which was given the name "Strachan's syndrome."

[22] Niacin is also required for the synthesis of the active forms of vitamin B3: nicotinamide adenine dinucleotide [NAD] and nicotinamide adenine dinucleotide phosphate [NADP]. [Pay attention:
we're going to have a test first thing tomorrow in class on what NAD
and NADF mean.]

levels. The particular importance to us is its reported assistance in **improving circulation** and in the proper functioning of the **nervous system**. Dr. Lark Lands, in her as yet unpublished book, *Positively Well: Living With HIV as a Chronic, Manageable Survival Disease,* mentions niacin favorably as one of the B complex members particularly helpful in **rebuilding the myelin sheath** around nerves of HIV patients afflicted with PN.

An early study observed that damage to the central nervous system can result from prolonged sleep deprivation as a consequence of **depletion** of nicotinic acid or niacin.[23] A later study found that treating rats in which diabetic neuropathy had been induced, with a derivative of nicotinic acid, had a **therapeutic effect** and that **motor nerve conduction velocity** (a marker of successful treatment as readers of *Toes and Soles* and *Toes and Woes* know) had improved.[24]

Good food sources for B3 include yeast, bran, rice, whole wheat, almonds, and peas.

A review panel under the auspices of the National Academy of Sciences' Institute of Medicine recently indicated that niacin could be used at doses up to 35 mg a day before side effects such as flushing were incurred. (The current RDI is 20 mg.) However some practitioners have prescribed the vitamin at levels as high as one to three grams a day for

---

[23] *Medical Hypotheses* (1991 Mar; 34(3): 275–77).
[24] *Journal of Diabetes Complications* (1995 Jul-Sep; 9(3): 133–39). Incidentally, there is one study that demonstrated peripheral neuropathy actually was made worse with the administration of niacin so caution is advisable in some cases. *Southern Medical Journal* (1998 Jul; 91(7): 667–68).

therapeutic purposes. Because of the risk of liver inflammation at dosages over one gram, however, medical supervision is particularly important at those high levels.[25]

Interactions occur principally with cholesterol-lowering drugs in the statin family or with alcohol if consumed excessively. In these cases people are particularly counseled not to take niacin except under a physician's supervision. Interactions are also said to occur with anticonvulsant drugs such as carbamazepine (Tegretol).

4. B5

Vitamin B5 or **pantothenic acid** is considered one of the best **energy enhancing** vitamins and is also valued for its **anti-inflammatory** properties. Similarly to B1, this vitamin is needed to make the neurotransmitter acetylcholine. Synthesis of cholesterol depends on pantothenic acid. The vitamin also activates the adrenal glands. A variation—**pantethine**—has been reported to lower blood levels of cholesterol and triglycerides.[26]

In a 1997 study at the Munchener Medizinische

---

[25] An article in *U.S. News & World Report* (April 16, 2001), pointed out that niacin has been used a long while to lower the risk of heart disease. The report said that at daily dosages where it is often administered—2000 mgs or more—many people experience flushing and nausea—plus the risk of liver damage. The report discussed a new form of niacin called "Niaspan," available only by prescription, which releases niacin into the blood stream at a controlled rate, thereby reducing the risk of adverse side effects.

[26] Technically pantethine is the stable structure of pantetheine, which is the biologially active form of pantothenic acid. Get it? If not we can try it backwards.

Wochenschrift in Germany, reported by the Life Extension Foundation, 28 out of 33 patients who had been treated solely with alpha-lipoic acid (more on that nutrient later) for PN showed further improvement when vitamin B5 was added to the treatment.

The best natural food sources for vitamin B5 are considered to be brewer's yeast, torulu (nutritional) yeast, calf liver, fish and shellfish, poultry, and soybeans. Peanuts, mushrooms, and split peas are supposed to be fairly good sources as well.

The RDI for pantothenic acid is 10 mg. For general health, though, it's been suggested that 100 to 200 milligrams per day might be appropriate. Therapeutic dosages are in the 600 to 1200 mg range. Toxicity is said not to occur below 10 *grams*. Symptoms beyond that level are reported to be occasional diarrhea and edema. No significant safety issues have been reported for pantothenic acid or pantethine when used with other medications.

5. B6

B6 or **pyridoxine** is important in manufacturing **prostaglandins**, which are oxygenated unsaturated cyclic fatty acids that have a variety of hormone-like actions such as assisting in the transport of oxygen in the blood stream. B6 is also needed for more than 100 enzymes involved in protein metabolism and for red blood cell metabolism. This vitamin is used as well for the conversion of tryptophan (an amino acid) to niacin (B3). Moreover, the nervous and immune systems require B6 to function efficiently.

A Japanese study considered the relationship of B6 deficiencies in 66 patients on chronic peritoneal (the peritoneum is the smooth membrane that contains the abdominal organs) dialysis, and peripheral neuropathy. The investigators found a direct correlation between the vitamin deficiencies and neuropathic symptoms, particularly with respect to the subjects who were elderly. Within one month after the administration of vitamin B6 supplementation, internal levels of pyridoxal phosphate had risen and sensory PN abnormalities had improved. The investigators seemed to go even further in their assessment of the results in concluding "if vitamin B6 deficiency is appropriately treated by oral supplementation, sensory abnormalities can be *eliminated* [emphasis added]." [27]

Another study (cited in the previous chapter) concluded that B6 supplementation was effective in "improving PPN [peripheral polyneuropathy] symptoms of various aetiologies," even though a deficiency could not be demonstrated in patients with chronic renal failure. [28]

Mention should again be made of the 1997 Tanzanian investigation reported in the previous section on B1. There clinicians had found superior outcomes in the treatment of diabetic neuropathy using therapeutic dosages of B1 and B6 compared with lower dosages. [29]

---

[27] *Advances in Peritoneal Dialysis* (2000; 16: 308–12). An earlier study found that elderly people tended to have "sub-optimal levels" of both riboflavin and B6 in spite of apparently adequate dietary intakes. *American Journal of Clinical Nutrition* (1998 Aug; 68(2): 389–95).

[28] *Nephrology, Dialysis, Transplantation* (2000 Sep; 15(9): 1410–13).

[29] *East African Medical Journal* (1997 Dec; 74 (12): 803–808).

In order for vitamins to be utilized by the body, they must first be converted into their active coenzyme forms. **Pyridoxal-5-Phosphate (PLP or P-5-P)** is considered the most **metabolically active** coenzyme form of vitamin B6. It is synthesized primarily in the liver from pyridoxine, with the help of enzymes that require vitamin B2, zinc, and magnesium for their activity.

The **sublingual** (under the tongue) administration of P-5-P is said in particular to help assure a higher degree of bioavailability of the vitamin to the body. This is because the substance is rapidly absorbed directly into the blood stream rather than passing through the digestive tract as is true with the usual pill-with-water routine. Sublingual absorption thereby avoids exposure to the dilutive effect of the gastric system and liver.

P-5-P supplementation is available in sublingual tablets from several suppliers. The tablets I have seen advertised usually contain 25 mg of the coenzymated substance, which yields about 17 mg of B6. The suggestion from those suppliers is one tablet daily or as recommended by one's health care professional.

Incidentally, **high dosages** of B6 can be **toxic** and can actually **cause** peripheral neuropathy.[30] (According to R. Andrew Sewell, M.D., at the Department of Neurology

---

[30] "Alcohol and Nutritional Neuropathies," by Laurence J. Kinsella, M.D. (1998 Neurobase Medline).

S.R. Snodgrass of the Department of Neurology at the University of Southern California School of Medicine, said in a paper entitled, "Vitamin Neurtoxicity," that "The only well-established human vitamin neurotoxic effects are those due to hypervitaminosis A (pseudotumor cerebri) and pyridoxine (sensory neuropathy). In each case, the *neurological effects of vitamin deficiency and vitamin excess are*

and Psychiatry, University of Massachusetts Medical School, the toxic effect of excessive pyridoxine consumed for an extended period of time on the dorsal root ganglions—sensory fibers in a spinal nerve root—causes a "pure sensory neuropathy.")

Most doctors think that up to 50 milligrams may be taken daily without concern. (The RDI is two milligrams.) In fact the general view seems to be that a definite PN risk does not usually occur until daily dosages exceed 200 milligrams. Apart from peripheral neuropathy, other health risks at that point include dizziness, nausea, and ataxia (a failure of muscular coordination). It should be noted that at least a few neurologists would limit the daily intake of B6 to 25 mg for people currently afflicted with PN.

Although vitamin B6 appears to be relatively safe when dosages do not exceed those indicated above, it is said to interact with the drug, levodopa. Particular caution should be used when these substances are taken together; consult a medical professional in such cases (as usual).

Vitamin B6 is found naturally in a wide variety of foods. Good sources include fortified breakfast cereals, fish—especially salmon and tuna, meats such as pork and chicken, bananas, beans, peanut butter, and many vegetables. A high protein diet reportedly increases the requirement for this nutrient.

---

similar. [Emphasis added]." *Molecular Neurobiology* (1992 Spring; 6(1): 41–73).

6. B12

Vitamin B12 is the name for a group of biological compounds essential to the body known as **cobalamins**. (The "cobal" in the name refers to the metal cobalt contained in B12.) This nutrient is needed to make DNA, the genetic material in all cells. In addition to contributing to the **metabolism of nerve tissue**, vitamin **B12** helps guard against stroke and heart disease and is said to contribute to relief from asthma, depression and low blood pressure.

Cobalamin is bound to protein in food and is released by hydrochloric acid in the stomach during digestion. Once released, B12 combines with a substance called intrinsic factor (IF) before it is absorbed into the bloodstream.[31]

B12 is thought to be one of the most effective members of the B complex for PNers. Dr. Sheldon Hendler, a noted expert in vitamin therapies, reports that in a series of 39 patients treated for neurologic symptoms related to B12 deficiency, all showed improvement from taking the nutrient. Other studies have demonstrated that aggressive B12 therapy eases pain from the nerve damage of diabetic neuropathy. The flip side of this is that deficiencies of the vitamin can directly lead to peripheral neuropathy. (An article in a 1996 issue of *Nutrition Reviews* reported that "vitamin B12 deficiency is linked to peripheral neuropathy in 40% of cases.")

The most common form of this vitamin is called **cyano-**

---

[31] An absence of intrinsic factor prevents normal absorption of B12 and results in pernicious anemia.

cobalamin while the more neurologically active is designated **methylcobalamin** or **methyl B12.** (Incidentally, urinary excretion of methylcobalamin is about one-third that of a similar dose of cyanocobalamin, indicating substantially greater tissue retention of the former.)

Investigators have linked many central and peripheral neurological disorders to a deficiency in methyl B12. (See, e.g., "Methylcobalamin: A Potential Breakthrough in Neurological Disease," *HealthWatch*, Winter 1999.) As indicated above, the reverse also has proven true, with **significant neurological benefits** demonstrated when methylcobalamin is made available to the body in adequate amounts.

Our bodies actually produce a small amount of this substance in the liver. However, much larger amounts of methylcobalamin are said to be required to correct neurological defects and also to neutralize a highly toxic substance produced in the body called **homocysteine.** This **amino acid** is linked to heart disease, stroke, and other problems.[32] A fairly recent study also indicated that high

---

[32] Studies released in February 2001, at a meeting of the American Stroke Association in Ft. Lauderdale, Florida, strengthened the case that elevated levels of homocysteine can lead to strokes. Dr. Peter J. Kelly of Massachusetts General Hospital in Boston, and his team, combined the results of 14 studies involving more than 11,000 patients. Together, they suggested that people with high levels of homocysteine have a 75 percent greater risk of stroke than do those with average levels. The analysis also showed that people who suffer strokes have average homocysteine levels that are 18 percent higher than those who do not. (No one knows precisely what the ideal homocysteine level is. However, doctors estimate that one-quarter of the U.S. population has elevated levels.)

homocysteine levels were directly associated with diabetic neuropathy.[33]

Homocysteine tends to accumulate in the body when methyl 12 becomes deficient. (As will be explained later, measuring this accumulation is one way of determining whether the body is sufficiently and efficiently supplied with B12.) If adequate quantities of methyl 12 and its synergistic cousin, **folic acid** or **folate**, are present, the body is then able to recycle the homocysteine to **methionine**. This substance in turn is further metabolized into the amino acid S-adenosyl-methionine or **SAMe**, which was discussed in *Toes and Soles*.

The importance of SAMe is that it is used by the body in a **methylation** process which helps, among other things, to **regulate neurotransmitters**—mentioned before as chemical substances in nerve cells which relay pain messages to the brain.[34] In a supplement form, SAMe is sometimes used as an antidepressant, or for osteoarthritis.

A good deal of the work involving methylcobalamin has been done in Japan, the only country where it could be

---

[33] *Diabetic Medicine* (2001 Mar; 18 (3): 185–92).

[34] In a 1998 article in the *Journal of Neurological Neuro-Psychiatry*, there is a discussion of the underlying mechanisms and causes of neuropathy, and the role of oxidation on the methyl transfer cycle which causes a deficiency of SAMe. This report indicates that SAMe supplementation may be helpful in the treatment of neuropathy.

An earlier paper—"The Biochemical Basis of Neuropathy in Cobalamin Deficiency"—stated that the pathogenesis of neuropathy associated with B12 deficiency is thought to be related to interference with the methylation reactions in the central nervous system. The paper describes a ratio between SAMe and its product, and says that if there is a fall of SAMe in the ratio, clinical signs of neuropathy are likely to emerge. *Baillieres-Clin-Haematol* (1995 Sep; 8 (3): 479–97).

fairly easily obtained (but with a prescription required) before 1998. Investigators there were reported in 1987 to have found that introducing a high concentration of methylcobalamin into **spinal fluid** was both highly effective and safe for treating the symptoms of diabetic neuropathy.[35]

A 1994 study went a step further and studied **nerve regeneration** in rats from ultra-high doses of methyl B12. The researchers concluded that the administration of 500 micrograms/kg daily resulted in a significant **enhancement** in **nerve fiber density**.[36] (The typical human equivalent would be about 40 *mg*—the RDI is 6 *mcg*!) Their conclusion was that very high doses of methyl B12 could be helpful in treating peripheral neuropathies.[37]

A 1999 investigation examined the effect of methylcobalamin given **intravenously**. Nine chronic hemodialysis patients with diabetic neuropathy were administered 500 mcg injections three times a week for six months. The investigators found that at the end of that period the patients' pain and *paresthesia* had lessened and that **sensory nerve conduction velocities** had shown significant improvement.[38]

Injecting vitamin B12 **intramuscularly**, in either the methylcobalamin or cyanocobalamin form, has been the

---

[35] *Clinical Therapy* (1987; 9(2): 183–92).

[36] *Journal of Neurological Science* (1994 April; 122(20): 140–43).

[37] This was echoed in the *Health Watch* article previously cited: "High doses of methylcobalamin are needed to regenerate neurons as well as the myelin sheath that protects nerve axons and peripheral nerves."

[38] *Internal Medicine* (1999 June; 38 (6): 472–75).

preferred method of administration for years for this nutrient. (B12 is used supplementally for a variety of health reasons, including cardiovascular problems, Alzheimer's disease, chronic fatigue syndrome, and sleep disorders.[39]) The belief has been that injections enhance absorption by the body more readily and provide speedy and direct availability.

Recently, however, it has been argued that the **sublingual** manner of taking this vitamin is just as effective as injections.[40] At the 28th World Congress of Hematology it was reported (*Reuters*, August 30, 2000) that Israeli investigators tested 18 patients with B12 deficiency. They found blood levels of B12 had increased to normal in all patients after only a few days following the sublingual ingestion of 1000 mcg of the vitamin twice a day. No side effects were reported.

A monograph in the *Alternative Medicine Review* main-

---

[39] The level of B12 decreases with age, and age-related deficiencies are associated with such impairments as hearing and memory loss. According to one researcher, "Vitamin B12 deficiency is estimated to affect 10–15% of people over the age of 60." *Annual Review of Nutrition* (1999; 19: 357–77). (Laurence J. Kinsella, M.D., maintains, though, that many more have no symptoms of deficiency.)

A study was conducted involving 61 patients with a mean age of 63 years who had gastric surgery as far back as 30 years, and 107 controls. The researchers found that 31 % of the surgery group had a B12 deficiency compared to 2% of the controls. The researchers recommended that if a deficiency is found in patients who have undergone gastric surgery, they be put on a program of lifelong vitamin B12 therapy. *Annals of Internal Medicine* (Mar 1996; 124 (5): 469–76).

[40] As mentioned before, this method permits the rapid absorption of substances directly into the blood stream rather than through the digestive tract as is true with the usual pill-with-water routine.

tained that there is no therapeutic advantage in any particular method: **orally, intramuscularly**, or **intravenously**.[41] (No mention or distinction was made between the usual oral method of taking a pill with water, or placing it under the tongue.)

A 1992 study concluded that **oral** administration of 500 mcg of methylcobalamin three times daily for three months, resulted in subjective improvement in burning sensations, numbness, loss of sensation, and muscle cramps. There was no indication whether or not the administration was sublingual.[42] A study reported in *Lancet* found that oral supplementation with 2000 mcg daily was *three times* as effective as intramuscular injections in increasing vitamin B12 levels in pernicious anemia patients! In this case the oral supplementation reportedly was *not* sublingual.[43]

Some of the more recent studies concerning methylcobalamin have involved dosages as high as 25–60 mg per day for adult humans. (Incidentally, the RDA is 2 *mcg*.) The *Alternative Medicine Review* monograph cited above maintains the appropriate dosage for "clinical effect" is 1500–6000 mcg (1.5 to 6 mg) daily. The author argues that there is no therapeutic advantage in exceeding this level. The *Cecil Textbook of Medicine* (21st Ed., 2000, W. B. Saunders Company), states that 1000 to 2000 mcg (1 to 2 mg) daily is the "treatment of choice for most patients."

---

[41] 1998 Dec; 3(6).
[42] *Clinical Neurology and Neurosurgery* (1992; 94: 105–111).
[43] Nov 1998; 352: 1721–22.

The author also says that hematological and neurological responses are the same whether oral or parenteral (injected) administration is used.

The 1999 *HealthWatch* article previously mentioned suggests that PNers using alpha-lipoic acid should **also take** at least 5 *mg* of sublingual methylcobalamin a day to make sure that the ALA would be bioavailable to the peripheral nerves

Since it may have taken a long time for the body's natural stores of B12 to become depleted where there is a deficiency (the liver is said to store 4 mg of the vitamin, normally representing a 3–6 year supply), it may similarly take some while for restoration to be achieved. Dr. Lark Lands, who advocates that regular doses of B12 be taken in the form of **injections** or **nasal gel**, says that it can take two to eight weeks (at least for AIDS patients) to return to normal B12 status if the deficiency is severe. She also warns that it is critical to replace depleted B12 as soon as possible. Laurence J. Kinsella, M.D., points out that the prognosis for recovery becomes bleaker the longer treatment with B12 is delayed. In fact many medical professionals believe that in the most advanced stage of B12 deficiency, any damage caused may not be reversible.

Dr. Lands mentioned a study by Dr. Martin David, Division of Geriatric Medicine, West Penn Hospital in Pittsburgh, where he found a very strong correlation between the duration of B12 "deficiency-induced cognitive symptoms" in the elderly and response to therapy with B12 injections. The best cognitive responses came from those who had been experiencing problems for less than six months. For those who had symptoms from six months to a year there was still a "fairly good response." He said that for those whose symptoms had lasted longer, even substantial supplementation with B12 did not make for improvement.

There seems to be some confusion concerning appropriate **testing** for B12 deficiency. Typically many doctors have relied on simply measuring **serum (blood)** levels. The problem with this approach is that it does not reveal whether the B12 present in the blood is **available** to and is being properly used by the body, or if "**malabsorption**" is possibly occurring.[44] More sophisticated tests, measuring the presence of elevated **methylmalonic acid**

---

[44] Food cobalamin malabsorption is emerging as a major cause of vitamin B12 deficiency according to Emmanuel Andrès, M.D., in his paper appropriately entitled, "Food Cobalamin Malabsorption: A Usual Cause of Vitamin B12 Deficiency." *Archives of Internal Medicine* (July 2000; 160: 2061–62).

Malabsorption can result from the lack of "intrinsic factor," a binding protein produced by cells within the stomach and required for the proper absorption of vitamin B12, as previously mentioned. Dr. Kinsella claims that it can also result from an inability to separate cobalamin from food because of inadequate gastric activity, as well as syndromes such as bacterial overgrowth and tapeworm infestation. See his article, "Alcohol and Nutritional Neuropathies." *Neurobase* (April 1999).

Iron deficiency causes anemia in up to 20% of patients with malabsorption by reducing the supply of hemoglobin, the oxygen transporting pigment of red blood cells. Since malabsorption reduces the supply of folates, the resulting folate deficiency will cause abnormal growth of the red blood cells. Vitamin B12 will also be less absorbed. Vitamin B12 deficiency occurs late, where it may take up to 5 years to deplete the body store of vitamin B12. It should be noted that vitamin B12 is the only vitamin where body stores can last that long.

(MMA) and **homocysteine (HCY)** levels—taken together—are considered better markers and more suggestive of the need for B12 supplementation.[45]

HCY levels are checked in a **blood test** and MMA in a **urine test**. If one or both indicate these levels are **too greatly elevated**, it may be *tentatively* assumed that the body is not well supplied with **available** B12. However, whether in fact the test results indicate a true B12 deficiency can only finally be determined after the fact by **re-testing** following the administration of B12 supplements, to see if there was an improvement (i.e., lowering) of HCY and MMA levels.

M. Dianne Delva, M.D., writing in the *Canadian Family Physician*, agrees that the **blood level** of cobalamin is an **unreliable indicator** of deficiency and that tissue levels of the vitamin may be quite low even if the blood levels are normal. She goes on to say that neurological disorders may occur at vitamin B12 levels just slightly lower than normal in the blood and considerably above the levels usually associated with anemia—a marker some medical professionals mistakenly use to determine B12 adequacy.[46]

The best natural sources for B12 are said to be organ meats, clams, oysters, beef, eggs, milk, chicken, and

---

[45] See, e.g., the excellent article, "Laboratory Diagnosis of Vitamin B12 and Folate Deficiency," Snow, *Archives of Internal Medicine,* Vol. 159, June 28, 1999. Where vitamin B12 deficiency occurs, utilization of folic acid is impaired. See the discussion in the section on folates.

[46] May 1997; 43: 917–22.

cheese.[47] In fact liver is considered to be the number one source, perhaps not surprising considering that, unlike the other water-soluble vitamins, B12 is stored in the human liver.

Daily maintenance dosage for general health is put by some authorities at 100 to 200 micrograms (mcg) although the RDI is only 6 mcg. For therapeutic purposes it is sometimes suggested that at least one mg (1000 mcg) be taken daily. (The *Cecil Textbook of Medicine* referred to above says that considering B12's safety profile, efficacy, and cost, "it is better to give too much than too little.") No upper limits for toxicity have been established. It has been suggested, though, that extremely large dosages could lead to or exacerbate acne—not the biggest problem most of us face (on our faces).

As to drug interactions, if you are taking medications that reduce stomach acid including H_2 blockers such as Zantac, or if you are exposed to nitrous oxide anesthesia, it is said you may need extra B12. As always, you should consult a medical professional with regard to these matters.

7. Biotin

This "vitamin" is also known as **vitamin H** or **coenzyme R** and is found primarily in the body's liver, kid-

---

[47] Although eggs are considered a good dietary source of B12, the vitamin present there is poorly absorbed due to the presence of binding proteins in egg whites and egg yolks. (Ball, *Bioavailability and Analysis,* 509.) This demonstrates there can be a significant difference between abundance of a vitamin in a diet and the body's ability to use it beneficially.

ney and muscle tissues. Biotin is essential for **cell growth** and **replication** through its role in the manufacture of the nucleic acids DNA and RNA, which make up the genetic material of the cell.

The RDI is 300 mcg. There is some evidence, however, that megadosages can be effective in improving nerve conduction and relieving PN pain. In a study performed at the University of Athens, subjects with PN were given 10 mg by intramuscular injection three times a week for six weeks, followed by 5 mg daily taken orally. Within four to eight weeks symptoms were reported to have decreased significantly (specifically painful muscle cramps, *paresthesias*, ability to stand, walk and climb stairs, and disappearance of restless leg syndrome in all patients) with no adverse side effects.[48] Dr. Lark Lands, who comments on the study, suggests that taking 10–15 mg of biotin daily, in conjunction with other B vitamins, might prove useful in improving nerve function.

Incidentally, neurological damage caused by long-

---

[48] *Biomed Pharmacother* (1990; 44 (10): 511–14).

An earlier study concerned 9 patients who had undergone chronic hemodialysis for 2–10 years and suffered from encephalopathy (dialysis dementia) as well as peripheral neuropathy. Ten mg of biotin was given daily in three doses for 1–4 years. Within 3 months there was a marked improvement in all patients in respect to disorientation, speech disorders, memory failure, jerks, flapping tremor, restless legs, *paresthesia,* and difficulties in walking. Based on the favorable outcomes from the biotin administration, the investigators recommended that biotin should be started early and regularly in any patient with advanced renal failure before severe neural or muscular lesions become manifest. The correlation of biotin with uremic neurologic disorders and the possible mechanism of its therapeutic action were also discussed. *Nephron* (1984; 36 (3): 183–86).

standing biotin deficiency has been thought by some to be irreversible. However a study was reported of a 15 year-old boy who had suffered "bilateral optic neuropathy" for five years. He also developed a "motor-type neuro-axonal" neuropathy in all limbs. Tests indicated that he suffered from severe biotin depletion. Following daily oral administration of 10 mg for a short period his "metabolic derangements subsided rapidly." Follow-up studies a year later showed "remarkable recovery" from the neuropathic conditions.[49]

Biotin is said to work closely with folic acid, pantothenic acid, and vitamin B12, and lessens the symptoms of pantothenic acid and zinc deficiencies. Deficiency of biotin itself is rare unless one eats large quantities of egg whites. Where it occurs, loss of appetite, anemia, fatigue, nausea, high blood sugar, and muscular pain are possible consequences.

This nutrient is widely distributed in foodstuffs, including liver, egg yolk, and green vegetables, but the amounts are small relative to other vitamins. People taking anti-seizure medications or large amounts of alcohol are said to need extra amounts.

Therapeutic dosages of biotin for those with conditions such as diabetes are reportedly as high as 7 to 15 *mg*. No upper limit for the nutrient has been determined and no adverse effects have been noted from high doses.

---

[49] *Neuropediatrics* (1993 Apr; 24 (2): 98–102).

8. Folate

Also referred to as **folic acid**, **folate** is said to rank number one in vitamin deficiency in North America. (The terms are sometimes used interchangeably but technically, folate is the natural nutrient found in foods and folic acid the synthetic form.) The nutrient is involved in a large number of **metabolic processes**, perhaps the most important being the **synthesis of DNA**.

DNA can be seriously damaged through attacks by free radicals so an adequate antioxidant status is essential to cell health. However, it is now becoming clear that antioxidants alone are not enough to protect our DNA; more and more research points to folate as being equally or perhaps even more important in ensuring proper DNA replication.

Folate is considered particularly helpful in the **maintenance of nerve cells.** Also the role of folate as a **methyl donor** interacting with B12 to create methylcobalamin, which is used in the re-methylation of homocysteine to methionine, has been previously mentioned.

In a paper entitled "Nutrition and Depression," the authors said that among patients with severe **folate deficiency**, peripheral neuropathy was one of the most common "**neuropsychiatric**" complications, following depression and dementia.[50]

Besides these three complications, deficiency some-

---

[50] Jonathan E. Alpert, M.D., Ph.D., Maurizio Fava, M.D., Harvard Medical School (1997).

times leads to anemia, constipation, and infections. Several medical conditions **increase the risk** of folate deficiency. Liver disease and kidney dialysis, which intensifies excretion (loss) of folic acid, are leading examples.

Similarly to B12 and biotin, folic acid is occasionally given intramuscularly by injection for PN. In these instances where it has been used therapeutically, folic acid reportedly has been administered in dosages of 1 *mg* or more (the RDI is 400 *mcg)*. It is recommended that supplementation of folate should include vitamin B12 so as not to mask an underlying B12 shortage. (The possibility of this masking is particularly worrisome among the elderly.[51]) Masking can occur because anemia might be alleviated by the folate but concomitant nerve degeneration as a result of B12 shortage will be undetected.

Good natural food sources are said to include legumes, liver, leafy green vegetables (in fact folate gets its name from the Latin word "folium" for leaf), beans, and nuts. In high dosages folic acid can possibly cause flatulence, nausea, and anorexia. The point at which toxicity may occur is said to be about 5 *mg*. The supplement should be used with caution in epileptics since folic acid can lower the seizure threshold.

---

[51] There are close interrelationships between B12 and folate. Vitamin B12 influences the storage, absorption, and utilization of folate for one thing. Further, as a deficiency of B12 progresses, the requirement for folate increases. However, increasing folic acid does not change the requirement for B12 even though anemia might be corrected. Permanent nerve damage might result if the B12 deficiency is not treated.

Oral pancreatic extracts (eg., pancrelipase or octreo-tide) can reduce folic acid absorption and it is recommended that the folic acid be given at different times from administration of these extracts. Estrogens, alcohol, chemotherapeutic drugs, sulfasalazine, barbiturates, and other anticonvulsants interfere with folic acid absorption and folate function.

9. Inositol

This nutrient, found **naturally** in the body, should perhaps be regarded as a distant relative rather than a direct family member of the B complex. It is present in all body tissues, with the highest levels in the heart and brain. Inositol is a constituent of **cell membranes** and plays a role in helping the liver process fats as well as contributing to the function of muscles and nerves. The nutrient works very closely with another B-complex vitamin, **choline,** discussed below.

Neurotransmitters such as serotonin and acetylcholine in the brain depend on inositol to function properly. Low levels of these neurotransmitters may result in **depression**; boosting inositol levels appears to be a promising treatment for that syndrome. Inositol's effect on depression led to a related study that concluded that it could reduce the frequency and severity of **panic attacks**.

Investigations concerning the administration of **myo-inositol** (a biologically active form of inositol) for peripheral neuropathy have been directed mainly to those with diabetes. In an early study, the nutrient was given twice a day—500 mg each time—to seven diabetic patients for two weeks. From the results the investigators concluded "myoinositol may be valuable in the treatment of diabetic neuropathy."[52]

The studies since have gone in different directions. A few years after the foregoing investigation, 28 young diabetics with short disease durations participated in a double-blind study by taking six grams of myoinositol or placebo daily for two months. The aim was to demonstrate a possible beneficial effect on "sub-clinical diabetic neuropathy." Measurement of vibratory perception threshold, motor and sensory conduction velocity, and amplitude of nerve potential—all markers of PN—did not disclose any beneficial effect from the myoinositol.[53] Yet another study, involving diabetic neuropathy induced in laboratory rats, found that nerve conduction velocity, which had decreased, was completely restored by the introduction of 1% dietary myoinositol.[54] In still another investigation, researchers at the University of Alabama found a statistically significant improvement in nerve function among diabetic patients placed on a diet high in inositol, including such high-inositol foods as cantaloupe, peanuts, grapefruit, and whole grains.[55] (Actually these foods supply a substance called phytic acid—inositol hexaphosphate, or IP6—which releases inositol when acted on by bacteria in the digestive tract.)

---

[52] *Lancet* (1978 Dec 16; 2(8103): 1282–84).
[53] *Acta Neurol Scand* (1983 Mar; 67(3): 164–72).
[54] *Diabetes* (1997 Feb; 46 (2): 301–06).
[55] No citation is available.

In some studies, decreased levels of inositol have been found in nerve cells of people with diabetes.[56] The investigators in these have concluded that the reduced levels, resulting from a build up of **sorbitol**, may be partially responsible for diabetic PN.[57] Again other studies have reached opposite conclusions, at least as to the relevance of inositol levels.[58]

Investigators in a Swedish study found that **nerve regeneration** positively correlated to **myoinositol** levels, with signs of "increased cluster density" at higher myoinositol levels.[59]

Dr. Robert Atkins has reported success in treating peripheral neuropathy with two to six grams of myoinositol daily. He notes that physicians at St. James Hospital in Leeds, England, have reported good results with smaller dosages.

---

[56] Also reduced levels of myoinositol have been observed in the sciatic nerves of rat models in which diabetic neuropathy has been induced. *Journal of Anatomy* (1999 Oct; 195 (Pt 3): 419–27).

[57] "Intracellular accumulation of sorbitol is most likely to cause depletion of other intracellular compounds including osmolytes such as myoinositol and taurine. . . which cause the clinical complications observed in diabetes, e.g., retinopathy, neuropathy. . . . *"Diabetes/Metabolism Research and Reviews* (2001 Sep; 17(5): 330–46).

[58] "Mean nerve levels of myoinositol were not decreased in the diabetic patients, with or without neuropathy, and were not associated with any of the neuropathological end points of diabetes. Our results indicate that myoinositol deficiency is not part of the pathogenesis of human diabetic neuropathy, as had been hypothesized." *New England Journal of Medicine* (1988 Sep 1; 319(9): 542–48). Confusion reigns; from the study noted in *Diabetes* cited above: "Dietary myoinositol supplementation. . . support[s] a role of myoinositol depletion in the genesis of early diabetic neuropathy."

[59] *Diabetic Medicine* (2000 Apr; 17(4): 259–68).

Most therapeutic dosages seem to be in the 1000–2000 mg daily range. (Some people take the active form, myo-inositol, as a supplement in one or two gram amounts daily to help them sleep better or to reduce nervous tension.) Experimentally, up to 18 grams daily have been tried for various conditions. Incidentally, caffeine-containing foods and beverages may create inositol shortage in the body.

As to natural sources, a study by R. S. Clements in the *American Journal of Clinical Nutrition* reported that:

> Since virtually no information is available concerning the myoinositol content of dietary constituents, we have measured the amount of this material present in 487 foods by gas-liquid chromatography. We observed that the greatest amounts of myoinositol were present in fruits, beans, grains, and nuts. Fresh vegetables and fruits were found to contain more myoinositol than did frozen, canned, or salt-free products.[60]

No serious ill effects or particular drug interactions have been reported for inositol where it is supplemented although high dosages may cause gastrointestinal upset, nausea, and diarrhea. A special precaution: even though it has been recommended for bipolar disorder, there is evidence to suggest inositol may trigger manic episodes in people with that condition.

In conclusion, based on the diversity of clinical results, one can only say the case for specially supplementing this B complex nutrient for PNers is less than overwhelming.

---

[60] 1980 Sep; 33(9): 1954–67.

10. Choline and Lecithin

Lecithin as sold in health stores contains phosphatidylcholine (generally referred to simply as PC—thankfully), a protector of cells in our nervous systems. PC itself is a source of choline which in turn forms yet another chemical in our bodies called acetylcholine. This latter chemical is an important neurotransmitter said to mediate emotions and behavior. Choline also acts like folate and SAMe to promote methylation (see the discussion in the section on vitamin B12).

There are indications lecithin and choline contribute to the production of **myelin,** the covering which protects nerves. There is also some evidence that these nutrients can be helpful in treating various neurological disorders such as Parkinson's disease, Alzheimer's, and Tourette syndrome.

For use as a supplement, lecithin is often manufactured from **soy.** In an interesting study performed at the Hadassah University Hospital in Jerusalem in 2000, investigators determined that soy-containing diets fed to rats in which neuropathic disorders had been induced, lessened the symptoms of the disorders. The investigators said there were implications from this study that warranted further investigations to determine the role of soy-containing diets for humans suffering chronic neuropathic pain.[61]

---

[61] *Anesthesia & Analgesia* (2001 Apr; 92 (4): 1029–34).

In a study reported in March 2002 to the American Pain Society, researchers at Johns Hopkins said that rats fed soy-based products

Ordinary lecithin contains about 10–20% PC. European products tend to have PC concentrated to about 90%. Based on those products, dosages as high as 5–10 grams taken three times daily have reportedly been used in studies for neurological conditions.

Lecithin is believed to be generally safe but people taking high dosages (three or more grams daily) sometimes experience minor side effects such as abdominal discomfort, diarrhea, and nausea. Maximum safe dosages have not been established. Lecithin is found in egg yolks, meat organs, green leafy vegetables, wheat germ, and as noted, in soy products.

Choline, which comes from lecithin, may also be taken directly as a supplement. For therapeutic purposes it is used anywhere from 500 to 1200 mg daily, the exact amount depending on the way the product is formulated to supply the active ingredient. The "adequate intake" for adult males is 550 mg per day and for females, 425 mg per day. (An RDI has not been established.) This nutrient is considered quite safe. The so-called "upper limit"—which is defined as the "highest daily intake over a prolonged period of time known to pose no risks to most members of a healthy population"—is 3.5 grams. (I saw another reference indicating choline could be used at up to 20 grams before toxicity would occur.) Side effects for

---

were better able to withstand heat applied to their injured paws, and had significantly less inflammation swelling, than did rats fed a milk-based diet. According to the report, the investigators believe their research could lead to "better options" for humans suffering chronic pain.

excessive intakes are about the same as from too much lecithin.

Before leaving the B complex, the special importance of these nutrients **individually** and **in combination** should be underscored. Even if you decide not to supplement a particular member of the complex individually (which as you will see later would be a mistake for most PNers, in my judgment), you should at least add a good B50 or B100 formulation to your dietary program.

Vitamin C

The scientific evidence is not as strong for vitamin C, also known as **ascorbic acid** or ascorbate, as for most of the members of the B complex in helping with neuropathy. Still there are studies and references "in the literature" which offer at least tangential support for its use here.

Vitamin C is considered the most popular vitamin supplement, certainly in the United States. One of its principal functions is to help the body **manufacture collagen**, an important protein for connective tissue, cartilage, and tendons. However its more prominent use is in the treatment of colds.

For our purposes, the most significant aspect to vitamin C is its potential as an **antioxidant.**[62] In addition to

---

[62] "These data [from a study concerning lipid peroxidation and cell killing and the administration of vitamins C and E] document the antioxidant function of the physiological level of cellular vitamin C and relate this function to protection against peroxidative cell injury." *Molecular Pharmacology* (1996 Oct; 50(4): 994–99).

the direct benefit it provides in fighting free radicals, vitamin C specifically complements the action of nutrients in the B complex in this regard. It also enhances the antioxidant effects of vitamin E, glutathione, and selenium. Moreover, vitamin C plays an important role in the manufacture of **neurotransmitters**.

Adequate levels of ascorbic acid are considered indispensable to good health in general. A National Health and Nutrition Examination Survey examined the vitamin C intake of over 11,000 people during a five-year period. Results showed that those in the high vitamin C intake group (greater than 50 mg daily) had a *48 per cent* lower chance of death from all causes in any period than those in the low intake group (less than 50 mg daily).

Studies performed at the University of Scranton and reported in *High-Speed Healing* (authored by the editors of *Prevention Magazine*) found that vitamin C can reduce the concentration of sorbitol, a type of sugar, in red blood cells and in this way protect against diabetic neuropathy.[63]

One study indicated that a combination of vitamin C with GLA (gamma-linolenic acid)—more on that later—was much more effective in treating peripheral neuropathy than GLA alone.[64]

A few studies or reports concerning medical conditions somewhat similar to peripheral neuropathy in terms of

---

[63] Other studies also have recognized that an intracellular accumulation of sorbitol contributes to the progression of diabetic complications [such as peripheral neuropathy] that are normalized with vitamin C supplementation. See, e.g., *Journal of the American College of Nutrition* (1994 Aug; 13(4): 344–50).

[64] *Diabetologia* (1996; 39: 1047–54).

physical distress indicate vitamin C can be used effectively for those conditions. One dealt with **reflex sympathetic dystrophy (RSD)**, an affliction that frequently causes persistent pain and difficulty of movement. In a double-blind investigation, either 500 mg of the vitamin or placebo was given daily to 123 individuals who had suffered wrist fractures, a frequent cause of RSD. After 50 days the treated group reported significantly fewer cases of RSD developing than did the placebo group.[65]

There are also anecdotal reports concerning the efficacy of vitamin C treatments for **restless legs syndrome**, a complication of neuropathy manifested by creeping, crawling sensations accompanied by motor restlessness, most often experienced at night.[66]

A Japanese study considered the effectiveness of treating a relatively rare syndrome called "Leber hereditary **optic neuropathy**" with vitamin A and vitamin C.[67] The investigators found that the administration of these two vitamins resulted in a "significantly shorter" visual recovery period for those given the vitamin therapy as contrasted with a control group which did not receive vitamins.[68]

Even if the evidence is not particularly strong for vita-

---

[65] *Lancet* (1999; 354: 2025–28).

[66] See p.151 of the *Natural Health Bible*, by Steven Bratman, M.D. (Prima Publishing 2000).

[67] LHON can cause loss of vision and is only passed on by women to their children, not by men. It is believed to be associated with neurological abnormalities in a manner somewhat similar to many of the more common neuropathies.

[68] *Journal of Neuro-ophthalmology* (2000 Sep; 20 (3): 166–70).

min C being especially beneficial in helping to treat PN, its marked **antioxidant capability** probably provides reason enough for PNers to use vitamin C on a regular basis in combination with other nutrients.[69]

Vitamin C is one of the vitamins that the body cannot manufacture but which must be obtained from food or supplements. Good natural sources include fresh fruits, especially berries and citrus, peppers, tomatoes, and cabbage.

· The RDA for vitamin C was long ago set at 60 mg daily; the RDI is the same. For therapeutic purposes practitioners suggest a level of 500 to 1000 mg (.5 to 1 gram) daily.

Toxicity is not considered a problem unless very large doses are ingested. Some consider that regular intakes of over 4 grams daily could present minor troubles such as nausea, diarrhea, with the possibility of kidney stones occurring if truly large dosages are taken over an extended period. It should be specially noted that large doses taken at the same time acetaminophen is used can pose the risk of liver damage.

It is possible to find vitamin C in many different forms, and various claims regarding efficacy or bioavailability

---

[69] Antioxidants such as vitamin C act to protect cells against the effects of **free radicals**, which are potentially damaging by-products of the body's metabolism as discussed earlier. Free radicals can cause cell damage that may contribute to the development of cardiovascular disease and cancer.

"Evidence supports that fruits and vegetables containing generous amounts of antioxidant nutrients are important for neurological function." *J Gerontol A Biol Sci Med Sci* (2000 Mar; 55(3): B144–51). A French study made the point that antioxidant defenses improved in elderly subjects with low doses of vitamins C and E. *Journal of the American College of Nutrition* (1997 Aug; 16 (4): 357–65).

have been put forward with respect to them. For instance, assertions are often made that **natural** ascorbic acid is superior to the **synthetic** product. However, Jane Higdon, R.N., Ph.D., a research associate at the Linus Pauling Institute, says that as assessed by at least two studies, there appears to be no clinically significant difference in the bioavailability and bioactivity between the two.[70] She also maintains that bioavailabilities appear equivalent whether the vitamin is taken in the form of powder, chewable tablets, or non-chewable tablets. Dashing some other views, she adds that bioavailability from slow-release preparations has not been found to be greater than that of plain ascorbic acid.

In her paper, "The Bioavailability of Different Forms of Vitamin C," (The Linus Pauling Institute, Oregon State University 2001), Ms. Higdon made some other interesting observations. She points out that **mineral salts** of ascorbic acid (mineral ascorbates) are **buffered**, and therefore, less acidic. However, she adds that "there appears to be little scientific research to support or refute the claim that mineral ascorbates are less irritating to the gas-

---

[70] One of the studies involved 12 males (6 smokers and 6 nonsmokers). The investigators found the bioavailability of synthetic ascorbic acid (powder administered in water) to be slightly superior to that of orange juice, based on blood levels of ascorbic acid, but not different based on ascorbic acid in white blood cells. *Journal of the American Dietetic Association* (1974; 64: 271–275).

The other study, of 68 male nonsmokers, found that ascorbic acid consumed as a component of cooked broccoli, orange juice, orange slices on the one hand, and synthetic ascorbic acid tablets on the other, were equally bioavailable, as measured by plasma (the liquid part of blood) ascorbic acid levels. *Journal of Nutrition* (1993; 123: 1054–61).

trointestinal tract." (Not everyone agrees and some nutritionists maintain that mineral ascorbates such as magnesium, calcium, potassium, and zinc, have a higher absorption rate. They also claim that combining mineral
ascorbates with some ascorbic acid permits a natural and
beneficial time-release of vitamin C.)

Ms. Higdon stresses that it is important to take into
consideration the dose of the mineral accompanying the
ascorbic acid when taking large doses of mineral ascorbates. For example, 1000 mg or 1 gram of **sodium ascorbate** contains 889 mg of ascorbic acid and 111 mg of
sodium. People on sodium-restricted diets may need to be
careful here. Pure **calcium ascorbate** provides 114 mg
of calcium per 1000 mg of ascorbic acid, she said, pointing out that total calcium intake should not exceed the
tolerable upper intake level of 2500 mg/day.

She points out in her paper that formulations sold as
Ester-C ascorbic acid contain mainly calcium ascorbate,
as well as small amounts of certain vitamin C metabolites,
and that manufacturers of these formulations claim that
these metabolites increase the bioavailability of the vitamin C in their products. A study they say that supports
their position, Ms. Higdon maintains, has not been published in a peer-reviewed journal. She refers on the other
hand to a small study of vitamin C bioavailability in 8
women and 1 man that found no difference between Ester-
C and commercially available ascorbic acid tablets with
respect to the absorption and excretion of vitamin C.[71]

---

[71] *Journal of the American Dietetic Association* (1994; 94: 779–81).
Nevertheless some proponents of Ester-C claim it is absorbed

Finally she did find possible merit in vitamin C compounded with **bioflavonoids**. (These are water-soluble plant pigments claimed to have good antioxidant qualities. Vitamin C-rich fruits and vegetables, especially citrus fruits, are often rich sources of bioflavonoids.) She mentions, for example, a study in which a natural citrus extract containing bioflavonoids was added to synthetic ascorbic acid. The investigators found that it was 35% more bioavailable than synthetic ascorbic administered without bioflavonoids.[72]

Incidentally, a number of manufacturers compound ascorbic acid with **rose hips**. These are the fruit of a rose remaining after the petals have fallen. Some claim rose hips have up to 60 times the Vitamin C of citrus fruit as well as bioflavonoids. (Ms. Higdon did not address this in her paper.)

300−400% more rapidly and retained longer in the body than ordinary forms of vitamin C. Jeffrey Bland, Ph. D., who has written extensively on nutritional matters, points to a couple of studies which do seem to indicate greater bioavailability for the Ester-C form. This would seem to be another area where more research is required.

[72] *American Journal of Clinical Nutrition* (1988; 48: 501–504). Undercutting the conclusion somewhat, though, was the fact that there was a greater proportion of bioflavonoids than found in typical commercial formulations.

In the study reported in the immediately preceding footnote, not only was there no special benefit found from the Ester-C nutrient, but no significant difference was found between the bioavailability of 500 mg of synthetic ascorbic acid without and that of a commercially available vitamin C preparation with added bioflavonoids

Vitamin E

Vitamin E is a fat-soluble nutrient that exists in a number of different forms. Each has its own special degree of **biological activity** or **bioavailability**, the measure of potency or functional use in the body. (This will be discussed in detail later). **Alpha-tocopherol** is the most active form in humans, and is a powerful biological **antioxidant**.[73]

A study reported in the journal, *Metabolism*, tested the effects of this vitamin on oxidative stress and free radical damage in Type 2 diabetic patients. The investigators found that **improving glycemic levels** (i.e., lowering blood sugar levels) with dietary changes and drugs lowered oxidative stress somewhat, but when these patients were supplemented with vitamin E for four weeks, oxidative stress and free radical damage were further reduced, "almost to the level of healthy people."[74]

Vitamin E exerts **enhanced** antioxidant effects in combination with other antioxidants including beta

---

[73] Other forms include beta-, delta-, and gamma-tocopherols, all of which occur in food. Commercially available vitamin E supplements contain primarily alpha-tocopherol, but researchers have found evidence that gamma-tocopherol also plays a crucial and complementary role in the body. In the April 1, 1997, issue of the *Proceedings of the National Academy of Sciences*, these researchers reported that gamma-tocopherol helps in "disarming destructive chemicals" (i.e., free radicals)—chemicals that alpha-tocopherol cannot completely neutralize.

[74] *Metabolism* (2000; 49: 160–62). Another study determined that "chronic administration" of high doses of vitamin E improved the cardiac autonomic nervous system of Type 2 diabetic patients by lowering oxidative stress levels. *American Journal of Clinical Nutrition* (2001; 73: 1052–57).

carotene, vitamin C, and selenium. It also regulates levels of vitamin A and may be required for the conversion of vitamin B12 to its active form. Additionally, vitamin E may reduce some of the symptoms of zinc deficiency.

Vitamin E is considered by many to be particularly important for **heart health**. In one investigation, dubbed CHAOS for Cambridge Heart Antioxidant Study and reported in *Toes and Soles*, 2002 men and women with artery narrowings were given either 400 or 800 IUs of vitamin E or a placebo daily. A statistical analysis following the study showed that vitamin E cut the risk of heart attack by more than half and the risk of a nonfatal heart attack by 77%.[75]

The particular importance of this vitamin to us is that it also sustains **normal neurological processes**, par-

---

[75] *Lancet* (1996 Mar 23; 347 (9004): 781–86). However that conclusion was seriously undercut by a later investigation—post *Toes and Soles*—in a study of 2545 women and 6996 men 55 years of age or older who were at high risk for cardiovascular events because they had cardiovascular disease or diabetes. The investigators found no significant differences in deaths or other cardiovascular outcomes between those on vitamin E and those on placebo: "In patients at high risk for cardiovascular events, treatment with vitamin E for a mean of 4.5 years had no apparent effect on cardiovascular outcomes." *New England Journal of Medicine* (2000 Jan 20; 342 (3): 154–60). (Imagine the thrill of the investigators at the Hamilton General Hospital in Ontario, Canada, demonstrating for the readers of the *New England Journal of Medicine*, how their English peers, reporting in the venerable, high-powered *Lancet*, had somehow gotten it all wrong.) Nevertheless there are many studies indicating cardiovascular benefit from vitamin E administration. Researchers are fairly certain that oxidative modification of LDL-cholesterol (sometimes called "bad" cholesterol) promotes blockages in coronary arteries that may lead to atherosclerosis and heart attacks. Vitamin E may help prevent or delay coronary heart disease by limiting the oxidation of LDL-cholesterol.

ticularly in its alpha-tocopherol form. A 1997 study reported in the American Family Physician suggested that a serious deficiency of vitamin E can have a profound effect on the central nervous system, leading to significant muscle weakness and visual field constriction.[76]

Earlier clinical studies demonstrated that low levels of vitamin E may lead to peripheral neuropathy.[77] The opposite was shown in a double-blind, randomized, placebo-controlled study of 21 subjects with diabetic neuropathy in Ankara, Turkey. The investigators found that nerve conduction had been improved significantly by the daily administration of 900 mg (sic) of vitamin E over a six-month period.[78]

Investigators in a Dutch study where "high doses" of vitamin E were given to rats in which diabetic neuropathy had been induced, indicated "nerve dysfunction had been prevented by 50%."[79]

A Korean study concluded that vitamin E-deficient neuropathy is reversible after four months of therapy (there was no indication of the dosage used).[80]

An interesting investigation in Italy indicated the administration of vitamin E to children before the age of

---

[76] 1997 Jan; 55 (1): 197–201: "Cystic fibrosis, chronic cholestatic liver disease, abetalipoproteinemia, short bowel syndrome, isolated vitamin E deficiency syndrome and other malabsorption syndromes all may cause varying degrees of neurologic deficits due to related vitamin deficiencies."

[77] See, e.g., *New England Journal of Medicine* (1987 Jul 30; 317 (5): 262–65).

[78] *Diabetes Care* (1998 Nov; 21 (11): 1915–18).

[79] *European Journal of Pharmacology* (1999 Jul 9; 376 (3): 217–22).

[80] *Archives of Physical and Medical Rehabilitation* (1999 Aug; 80(8): 964–67).

three could prevent or reverse neuropathies that might otherwise result from certain liver diseases.[81]

Vitamin E deficiency is generally quite rare in humans. This is because of the wide range of foods in which it is found, and the vitamin's widespread distribution throughout the body. An extended period of dietary insufficiency would be required before meaningful depletion occurs.

Vegetable oils, nuts, and green leafy vegetables are the main dietary sources of vitamin E. Fortified cereals are also an important source in the United States. If vitamin E is to be supplemented, many nutritionists recommend that the natural rather than the synthetic form be used. The former is called **d-alpha tocopherol**, while synthetic vitamin E is called **dl-alpha tocopherol**. Because much of the alpha-tocopherol in the synthetic vitamin is inactive, some nutritionists claim about twice as much is required to obtain the same effect as from the natural form.[82]

Vitamin E is formulated and sold as either **tocopherol**, or as **tocopheryl** followed by the name of whatever is attached to it, as in "tocopheryl acetate." In each case the tocopherol, or tocopheryl-with-attached name, is preceded by either d- or dl- to indicate whether it is natural or synthetic. Plain tocopherol may be absorbed a little better while tocopheryl-with-attached names have a slightly better shelf life. In **health food stores**, the most

---

[81] *Acta Vitaminologica Et Enzymologica* (1985; 7 Suppl 33–43).
[82] An early study, though, would shave the advantage, where the natural form was found to be 1.3 times as effective as the synthetic. *International Journal of Vitamin Nutrition Research* (1982; 52: 351–70).

common forms of vitamin E are d-alpha tocopherol and d-alpha tocopheryl **acetate** or **succinate**. Although the succinate form is slightly weaker than the acetate form, more milligrams of the succinate form are added to supplements to compensate for this small difference in potency. Therefore, 400 IU of either form should have equivalent potency.

The current RDI for vitamin E is 30 IUs, or 20 mg.[83] As noted in *Toes and Soles*, many practitioners suggest the nutrient be taken in doses of 400–800 IUs daily. A study of high doses in the treatment of neurological disorders in the elderly concluded that oral intakes of up to 2000 IUs daily were relatively safe for periods of up to two years. The investigators went on to say that "the safety and efficacy of supplemental vitamin E" over longer periods "had not been adequately explored."[84] The National Institute of Medicine has set an "upper tolerable intake level" for vitamin E at 1000 mg (1500 IU) for any form of supplementary alpha-tocopherol per day. Upper tolerable intake levels "represent the maximum intake of a nutrient that is likely to pose no risk of adverse health effects in almost all individuals in the general population."

---

[83] Vitamin E values have historically been given in International Units, or IUs. In a 1997 Dietary Reference Intake report, values were restated so that 15 mg is defined now as the equivalent of 22 IUs of natural vitamin E or 33 IUs of the synthetic form. The assumption made here on dosage is that the vitamin is taken is the natural form (d-alpha-tocopherol).

[84] *American Journal of Clinical Nutrition* (1999 Nov; 70(5): 793–801).

Vitamin E does exert a "**blood thinning**" effect that could possibly lead to problems in some situations. There is a particular concern if it is combined with medications that also thin the blood such as Coumadin (warfarin), heparin, and Trental (pentoxifylline). There is also said to be some concern that vitamin E could interact with herbs possessing a mild blood-thinning effect such as ginkgo biloba (discussed later).

Individuals wishing to take vitamin E are advised that it is especially important for them to consult their physician if taking oral hypoglycemic medications. There is also some question about vitamin E being taken at the same time that standard chemotherapy drugs are used since those drugs work in part by creating free radicals that destroy cancer cells; antioxidants such as vitamin E might interfere with this process, according to that reasoning.

In spite of these stated concerns, vitamin E is considered by some to be among the safest of the commonly ingested, fat-soluble vitamins.

"Vitamin Neuropathies"

For those PNers anxious to determine if their neuropathy happened to have been caused by a particular vitamin deficiency or a vitamin overload, the following discussion on etiological "clues" might be of interest. (Be forewarned, though, that the material is quite technical and written in "medicalese.")

As always, you should consult with your doctor who

can go into greater depth on these matters with you if you wish to pursue them. This discussion appeared in a paper entitled "Nutritional Neuropathy," authored by R. Andrew Sewell, M.D., and Lawrence D. Recht, M.D.[85]:

- Mouth: Glossitis suggests cyanocobalamin (vitamin B-12) deficiency; glossitis and cheilosis suggest pyridoxine (vitamin B-6) deficiency; gingivitis, stomatitis, and glossitis point to niacin (vitamin B-3) deficiency.
- Skin: Nasolabial seborrhea suggests pyridoxine (vitamin B-6) deficiency; a pellagrous skin rash niacin (vitamin B-3) deficiency; and hyperpigmentation a cobalamin (vitamin B-12) deficiency.
- Cardiovascular: CHF suggests thiamine (vitamin B-1) deficiency.
- Hematologic: A megaloblastic anemia suggests a cobalamin (vitamin B-12) or folate deficiency; a hypochromic anemia is usually iron deficiency but can also represent a pyridoxine vitamin (B-6) deficiency.
- Specific syndromes include the following:
  - Alcohol neuropathy: This is characterized by decreased pain and temperature sensation in a stocking-glove distribution, distal muscle weakness and atrophy (legs worse than arms) with stasis pigmentation and plantar ulcerations, wrist and foot drop, hyporeflexia with absent Achilles reflex, and an antalgic gait. The skin may be dry and scaly with rhinophyma (alcohol nose). Hepatomegaly, jaundice, or ascites may result from concurrent liver dysfunction. Alcohol neuropathy is frequently associated with entrapment or pressure neuropathies, particularly ulnar and peroneal,

---

[85] *EMedicine Journal*, Oct. 23, 2001, Vol. 2, No. 10. Permission from Dr. Sewell to set this material forth here is gratefully acknowledged.

which may be superimposed on the polyneuropathy. Charcot joints and Wernicke-Korsakoff syndrome may also be present.

○ Thiamine (vitamin B-1) deficiency: About 70%
have a polyneuropathy; of those 20% are motor
only, 50% motor-sensory, and 30% sensory only.
It is both subchronic and chronic; presentation
includes paresthesias and numbness, fasciculations and cramps, followed by dorsiflexor weakness with a steppage gait, and finally bilateral
lower extremity paraplegia develops. Thirty percent will manifest spread of the neuropathy to the
proximal muscles of pelvic girdle, trunk, and upper extremities.

The patellar and Achilles tendon reflexes will be
decreased. Cranial nerve manifestations include
retrobulbar optic neuropathy, hoarseness, dys-
phagia, and tachycardia from vagal involvement
and even bilateral facial paralysis in some cases.
Rarely, an acute paraplegic form presents with anorexia and vomiting, then in a day or two, a rapidly
progressive paralysis ascends from legs to arms
and shoulder girdle. Death follows within 2 days
from cardiac insufficiency.

○ Niacin (vitamin B-3) deficiency: Patients present
with decreased proprioception and vibratory sense,
weakness in legs with some fasciculations and
cramping, Babinski reflexes—equivocal or positive. Paresis is rare, deep tendon reflexes are decreased in 10–20% but increased in most. Simul-
taneous psychiatric disorders, extrapyramidal
symptoms, cranial nerve dysfunctions, and sei-
zures ultimately result.

○ Pyridoxine (vitamin B-6) deficiency: Presentation
includes seborrheic dermatitis, cheilosis, glossitis,
nausea, vomiting, weakness, and dizziness. Neuro-

logical exam shows decreased proprioception and vibration sense with spared pain and temperature sensations; normal strength; decreased or absent Achilles reflex and decreased patellar reflex. Ataxia if present is sensory.

○ Pyridoxine toxicity also can cause a neuropathy: Acute high dose (180 g) intoxication causes a sensory neuronopathy. Clinical manifestations include diffuse paresthesias, proximal and distal sensory loss, sensory ataxia, and autonomic dysfunction. Recovery tends to be poor. Chronic low doses (0.2–10 g/d) cause a milder distal sensory neuropathy, which presents with distal paresthesias and numbness. Recovery is usually good once pyridoxine is stopped.

○ Folate deficiency: Patients present with subacute combined degeneration, sensorimotor polyneuropathy, and dementia.

○ Cyanocobalamin (vitamin B-12) deficiency: Presentation includes a number of neurological findings, they are as follows:

  ▪ Corticospinal tract abnormalities—Spasticity; 50% lack Achilles reflex; some have no patellar reflex; bilateral positive Babinski; hyperreflexia is rare

  ▪ Posterior column abnormalities—Decreased vibration, temperature, and proprioception (lower extremities); sensory ataxia; positive Romberg sign in later stages

  ▪ Peripheral neuropathy—Moderate to severe, with muscular atrophy and weakness in later stages

  ▪ Behavioral and personality changes, particularly depression

○ Nutritional amblyopia: Patients present with decreased visual acuity and sometimes bilateral field defects with central or cecocentral scotomas. Early on, the optic discs show no change or papillitis on funduscopic exam; later the discs become pallid.

○ Nutritional sensorineural deafness: Presentation includes mild-to-moderate unilateral or bilateral hearing loss.

The "Nutritional Neuropathy" paper later suggests the tests that should be performed if "physical" examination and "history" are unrevealing:

- Check CBC, urine analysis (U/A), thyroid-stimulating hormone (TSH), glucose, renal and hepatic functions, vitamin B-12 level, ESR, and serum protein electrophoresis, then order other tests as needed. Electrophysiology can confirm the impression of polyneuropathy but will rarely provide the diagnosis.

    ○ Alcohol neuropathy: CBC may show low platelets and a megaloblastic anemia from decreased folate. [*Dr. Kinsella, commented to me with regard to this statement, that the problem may be due to direct toxicity from the alcohol and not necessarily due to folate deficiency.*]

    ○ Thiamine (vitamin B-1) deficiency: A serum thiamine (vitamin B-1) level is actually not a good index because it responds quickly to dietary supplementation and is a poor indicator of total body stores. Urinary excretion <65 mg/g creatinine is abnormal. Pyruvate levels >1 mg/dL is a reliable indicator of deficiency. The best test is an erythrocyte transketolase activity (<0.017 U/dL). [*Dr. Kinsella would modify the foregoing two sentences to read as follows: "Elevations of lactate and Pyruvate (levels >1 mg/dL) may be more reliable indicators of deficiency. A better test is an erythrocyte*

transketolase activity level following stimulation with thiamine pyrophosphate (the TPP effect)]
- Pyridoxine (vitamin B-6) deficiency: CBC shows a microcytic hypochromic anemia with normal iron levels. The serum pyridoxine levels are < 25 mg/mL. A tryptophan loading test (less commonly performed) reveals urinary xanthurenic acid excretion >50 mg/day.
- Folate deficiency: Serum folate levels are low.
- Niacin (vitamin B-3) deficiency: Urinary excretion of N-methylnicotinamide + N-methyl-6-pyridone-3-carboxamide is <2 mg, or urinary excretion of N-methylnicotinamide is <0.5 mg/g creatinine. It is also possible to perform a "stress test" by giving 10 mg niacin and 100 mg tryptophan; if urinary excretion of niacin metabolites is <3 mg, then a deficiency exists.
- Cyanocobalamin (vitamin B-12) deficiency: The CBC may show MCV >110 (a macrocytic anemia), anisocytosis, poikilocytosis, and large oval erythrocytes with a decreased reticulocyte count, leukocytes and platelets, but the neuropathy may precede any hematologic abnormalities. The serum cobalamin may be normal even with a tissue cobalamin (vitamin B-12) deficit. Serum homocysteine and methylmalonic acid are elevated, as is urinary methylmalonic acid excretion. Serum holo-transcobalamin II is deficient. Intrinsic factor antibodies are specific for pernicious anemia but not very sensitive (40% negative). The Schilling test, although classic, is rarely used now.
- Pantothenic acid deficiency: Excretion is <1 mg per day.
- Alpha-tocopherol (vitamin E) deficiency: Serum alpha-tocopherol (vitamin E) level is low; CBC shows acanthocytes.

○ Hypophosphatemia: Serum phosphate level is <1 mg/dL.

Imaging Studies:

• Imaging studies are generally not useful.
• Radiography of chronic peripheral neuropathies is often consistent with the picture of a diabetic foot.

Other Tests:

• Axonal loss manifests as a mild slowing of the nerve conduction velocity (NCV) with a disproportionate loss of amplitude. Demyelination, on the other hand, shows mild loss of amplitude with a disproportionate slowing of the NCV. In affected motor fibers, electromyography (EMG) shows fibrillations, positive sharp waves, and decreased motor unit potentials. EMG and NCV are useful to assess the degree of damage and monitor the progression of the neuropathy.
• Thiamine (vitamin B-1) deficiency: EMG and nerve conduction studies reveal a generalized axonal sensorimotor polyneuropathy with denervation of the distal lower extremity musculature; at times there may be some subtle demyelinating features present.
• Niacin (vitamin B-3): EMG and NCV show demyelination in mild cases and axonal degeneration in severe cases.
• Alpha-tocopherol (vitamin E) deficiency: Peripheral nerve conduction studies are normal. Sensory evoked potentials are low or absent. Somatosensory evoked potentials show a delay in central conduction. EMG is normal.
• Sensorineural hearing loss: Audiometry shows high-tone hearing loss.
• Alcohol: CSF protein on lumbar puncture is normal or slightly elevated.

Chapter 3

Minerals

Minerals are originally extracted from soil by plants but are labeled **inorganic nutrients** because they contain no carbon. Similarly to vitamins, many function as coenzymes, acting as catalysts for biologic reactions such as muscle response, digestion, and the transmission of messages through the nervous system.

Of the 60 minerals found in the body, only about a third are considered **essential** to human nutrition (accounting for approximately five pounds of the average person's weight). As with vitamins, essential in this sense means those that cannot be produced by the body but must be supplied by the diet or supplements.

Minerals recognized as essential are further classified either as **major minerals** or **trace minerals**. These designations do not necessarily reflect the relative importance of the minerals but rather the fact that, according to some classifiers (in rather a homespun way of looking at things), major minerals are present in the body in amounts greater than a teaspoon, while trace minerals total less than a teaspoon. Others would attempt a more precise delineation (after all, was the teaspoon level or heaping?) and say that, at least in so far as supplementation is concerned, major minerals are measured in milligrams or grams while trace minerals are measured in micrograms.[1] Regardless of how defined or measured, deficiencies of either major or trace essential minerals can have equally devastating health consequences.

The particular minerals that are most important to PNers are thought to be chromium, magnesium, selenium, and zinc, and they are all covered in this chapter. Another mineral not generally regarded as a nutrient is also briefly discussed here. You will see that this substance—lithium—has both potential beneficial as well as possible detrimental effects.

Chromium

Chromium is a trace mineral essential for normal **sugar and fat metabolism**. It works with insulin to move glucose into cells where it can be used to generate energy. Chromium also acts with insulin to stimulate **protein synthesis**. (Optimal chromium intake appears to decrease the amount of insulin needed to maintain

---

[1] The major minerals are said to include calcium, chloride, magnesium, phosphorus, potassium, sodium, and sulfur. The trace minerals include chromium, cobalt, copper, fluoride, iodine, iron, manganese, molybdenum, nickel, selenium, silicon, vanadium, and zinc. (Note that zinc proves the exception to the rule and is measured in milligrams rather than micrograms.)

normal blood sugar.) This mineral occurs throughout the body with highest concentrations in the liver, kidney, spleen, and bone.

Many otherwise good sources of chromium, such as whole wheat, are depleted of this important mineral during processing. Some medical professionals believe that inadequate intake of chromium may be one of the causes of the rising rates of adult-onset diabetes.

There is increasing appreciation of the role chromium plays in treating peripheral neuropathy. Doctors at the Department of Medicine, St. Michael's Hospital, in Ontario, Canada, found in 1996 that the infusion of 250 micrograms of **trivalent chromium**[2] daily into a patient who had peripheral neuropathy of the axonal type and was glucose intolerant, resulted in clinical remission that was marked 4 days after starting the infusion. Normalization of nerve conduction occurred within 3 weeks of the initial study.[3]

The new *Merck Manual of Diagnosis and Therapy* (17th Ed., Section 1, Chapter 4), reports a study of four patients with **glucose intolerance** and peripheral neuropathy. Three responded positively with doses of 150 to 250 mcg of trivalent chromium, with both a reduction in PN and an increase in glucose tolerance.

---

[2] Nutritional chromium is "trivalent chromium." The life-threatening chromium that was the subject of the Erin Brockovich film is known as "hexavalent chromium." (The film even makes this distinction, identifying the pollutant as hexavalent chromium.) Trivalent and hexavalent are chemical terms that refer to the net electronic charges of the two chromium molecules (hexavalent, +6; trivalent, +3).

[3] *J Parenter Enteral Nutr* (1996 Mar-Apr; 20 (2): 123–27).

Diabetes Metabolism refers to a study in which a patient with "severe neuropathy and glucose intolerance," had been on "total parenteral [by injection] nutrition," receiving currently recommended levels of chromium. The neuropathy and glucose intolerance reportedly were reversed by additional chromium supplementation.[4] Dr. Khursheed N. Jeejeebhoy, of the University of Toronto Medical Center, in a review of safety and health benefits of chromium, reported that in one of his patients who had not been taking supplements, progressive neuropathy had developed and that the mineral was markedly depleted in tissues at autopsy.[5]

A study in the *Journal of the American College of Nutrition* concluded that although 200 mcg of chromium daily was adequate for those who are mildly glucose intolerant, people with "more overt impairments" require higher dosages.[6] Specifically, a daily intake of 8 mcg per kg body weight was mentioned. This would be equal to about 544 mcg for a person weighing 150 pounds.

Another study acknowledged that impaired microcirculatory perfusion[7] appears to be central to the origin of neuropathy in diabetics. The associated dysfunctions, ac-

---

[4] 2000 Feb; 26(1): 22–7.

[5] Jeejeebhoy, K N. "The Role of Chromium in Nutrition and Therapeutics and As a Potential Toxin," *Nutrition Review* (1999; 57 (11): 329–35).

[6] *Journal of the American College of Nutrition* (1998 Dec; 17(6): 548–55).

[7] The microcirculation system consists of blood vessels such as capillaries with a diameter of less than 300 micrometers. Peripheral neuropathy is sometimes associated with a lack of blood circulation or perfusion to the nerve cells.

cording to the investigators, could be addressed with a supplementation program that includes high-dose antioxidants, fish oil, gamma-linolenic acid, **chromium**, arginine, and carnitine.[8]

However there are still some who question—or at least need more convincing of—dietary supplementation of chromium being necessary for those with diabetes. For example at a workshop held by the Office of Dietary Supplements at the National Institutes of Health in November 1999, it was said:

> The overriding question left to the committee was what is the best way to derive further information to determine whether a deficient chromium status plays a role in the incidence of diabetes in this country. Most perplexing is the fact that we do not yet have a good measure of chromium status, we cannot measure or assess deficiency in people, and we have not developed satisfactory animal models that can be extrapolated to humans. Hence, it becomes evident that the development of appropriate and sensitive biomarkers and outcomes measures are pivotal prior to initiation of formal clinical intervention studies. *It is clear that, for the general public, current data do not warrant routine use of chromium supplements, whose risk-benefit function has not yet been adequately characterized.* [Emphasis added]

Brewer's yeast and calf liver are the best natural sources for chromium. Vegetable oil and whole grain cereal are also considered good sources. Processing foods

---

[8] *Medical Hypotheses* (1998 May; 50(5): 435–49).

with stainless steel equipment may increase their chromium concentration, especially if the foods are acidic. In addition, there are differences in bioavailability and biological activity of the different complexes found in foods.

The RDI for chromium is 120 mcg daily. For those who decide to use the nutrient in supplemental form, the usual range seems to be 200 to 400 mcg per day. Therapeutic use extends up to 1000 mcg (1 mg) daily.

According to some reports, **chromium picolinate** is a better supplementation choice than chromium chloride because the former is said to be more readily available for use in the body. Reports by purveyors of the chromium picolinate form claim, in fact, that it is absorbed 7 times more efficiently than chromium from chromium chloride.[9] However, some questions have been raised as to its safety. Researchers at Northern Arizona University have questioned the use of chromium picolinate and suggested the possibility that it could lead to cancer. Specifically they point to a study where chromosomal damage was induced by chromium picolinate salt in hamster ovary egg germ cells, raising in their minds the possibility of "mutagenesis and carcinogenesis." The manufacturer of the compound violently disagrees, though, contending the dosages used in the animal study were way out of proportion to

---

[9] According to the Chromium Information Bureau, "The picolinate is complexed to the chromium and that makes it absorbed and used by the body more easily than other chromium forms. Why, we don't really know yet, but when given to humans and compared with chromium polynicotinate or chromium chloride, chromium picolinate is usually the most well utilized form."

what a human being would take. The jury is still out on this as of the time this was written.[10]

Putting aside the picolinate study, side effects from the ingestion of chromium are quite rare. According to *Modern Nutrition in Health and Disease,*[11] a leading nutrition reference book, "Trivalent (nutritional) chromium has such a low order of toxicity that deleterious (harmful) effects from excessive intake of this form of chromium do not occur readily. Trivalent chromium becomes toxic only at extremely high amounts—chromium then acts as a gastric irritant rather than as a toxic element interfering with essential metabolism or biochemistry." There is one report, though, of kidney damage to a person who took 1200 to 2400 mcg daily for several months. In another report as little as 600 mcg for 6 weeks was said to have caused damage.

If calcium carbonate supplements or antacids are being used, one may need extra chromium. Also, medical professionals say that chromium supplements and doses of those other substances should be separated by at least two hours so they won't interfere with chromium's absorption.

Magnesium

Magnesium is necessary for **nerve conduction** and for the **anaerobic breakdown** of **glucose**. The mineral

---

[10] There is no doubt, however, where the UC Berkeley Wellness Letter, in its June 1999 issue, stood: "Nobody should take chromium picolinate, especially not young people." Period.

[11] Shils, Olson and Shike, eds., 9th edition (January 1999 Lippincott, Williams & Wilkins).

is also vital for thiamin, vitamin C, and pyridoxine metabolism. Magnesium is needed, in fact, for more than 300 biochemical reactions in the body. It also helps keep heart rhythm steady, bones strong, and is involved in protein synthesis.

About half of the body's magnesium supply is found inside cells of tissues and organs, and half is combined with calcium and phosphorus in bone. Only one percent of the magnesium is found in blood. The body constantly strives to keep blood levels of magnesium constant.

This nutrient has sometimes been called "nature's calcium channel blocker," referring to magnesium's ability to impede calcium from entering muscle and heart cells. (Some prescription medicines work the same way although much more powerfully.) This blocking action could be the basis for magnesium's effects on migraine headaches and high blood pressure.

A recent study reported that magnesium deficiency increases susceptibility to the physiologic damage produced by stress, and that administration of the mineral has a protective effect against migraine and "transient ischemic" attacks. The author of the study concluded that:

"Mg [magnesium] ions have nutritional and pharmacologic actions that protect against the neurotoxicity of agents as diverse as environmental noise, sympathornimetic amines and physical trauma. Mg deficiency, even when mild, increases susceptibility to various types of neurologic and psychological stressors in rodents, healthy human subjects and diverse groups of patients. Repletion of deficiency reverses this increased stress sensitivity, and pharmacologic loading of Mg salts orally or parenterally induces resistance to neuropsychologic stressors." [12]

This mineral may be especially important for those with diabetes and diabetic neuropathy.[13] A recent paper reviewed a study of 35,988 older women who were initially free of diabetes. Of these, 1141 developed Type 2 diabetes within six years. The study determined that although dietary fiber intake led to the lowest chance to contract diabetes, the strongest **protective effect** was observed for magnesium consumption. Women who had consumed 332 mg of magnesium daily cut their risk of developing diabetes in half compared with women who consumed less than 242 mg daily.[14]

A few practitioners have found that magnesium deficiencies either cause peripheral neuropathy or are associated with PN. For example in a study of 128 patients with Type 2 diabetes conducted at the Department of Medicine, Bahia Federal University Medical School, Brazil, magnesium levels were found to be significantly lower in patients with peripheral neuropathy than in those in a control group.[15]

In a study conducted in Mexico, 33 out-patients with

---

[12] From a paper entitled "Magnesium, Stress and Neuropsychiatric Disorders," by Leo Galland, M.D., Director of the Foundation for Integrated Medicine at the Great Smokies Diagnostic Laboratory, Asheville, N.C., USA.

[13] Also for those with HIV infections. Dr. Lark Lands points out that in HIV patients, magnesium can be lost from their bodies as a result of infections and that any additional infections can greatly increase the likelihood of a magnesium deficiency.

[14] *American Journal of Clinical Nutrition* (2000 Apr; 71 (4): 921–30).

[15] *Diabetes Care* (1998 May; 21 (5): 682–86).

Type 2 diabetes and foot ulcers (16 women and 17 men) were compared with a control group of 66 out-patients with Type 2 diabetes without foot ulcers (35 women and 31 men), matched by age, diabetes duration, and glycemia. The investigators found that subjects with foot ulceration had lower serum magnesium levels than those in the control group and concluded magnesium depletion had led to peripheral neuropathies which then contributed to the foot ulcerations.[16]

Dr. Sally Stroud of the Houston Immunological Institute in Texas has found magnesium supplements help correct some neuropathies. In patients with decreased serum magnesium levels, she reports intravenous supplementation followed by oral augmentation decreased neuropathic sensations and the use of pain medications.

Michael Murray, N.D., the author of *A Textbook of Natural Medicine* and the *Encyclopedia of Natural Medicine*, advises patients that vitamin B6 and magnesium offer significant protection against the development of diabetic neuropathy and "offers some benefit in improving nerve function as well."

Jon Kaiser, M.D., in his book, *Healing HIV*,[17] in the chapter "Preventing and Treating Neuropathy," suggests calcium 500 mg, **magnesium** 250 mg, and vitamin B6 100 mg, twice a day for AIDS patients. If neuropathy has already been established he increases the dose of vitamin B6 to 200 mg twice a day, leaving the other levels the same. Dr. Kaiser noted that while improvement can occur

---

[16] *Archives of Medical Research* (2001 Jul-Aug; 32 (4): 300–303).
[17] *Health First Press*, 1998.

quickly, in some cases it may take several months before there is a noticeable change.[18]

Other doctors have also suggested adding 200 to 400 milligrams of supplemental magnesium daily to one's diet. (The RDI is 400 mg.) Therapeutic dosages can be in the 600 mg daily range. Dr. Mildred Seelig, a well-known magnesium researcher, would go further and reportedly has recommended a daily intake of 6 to 10 mg per kg of body weight per day for optimal health. As a matter of fact, because deficiencies are so common with this mineral, some medical professionals think it is probably reasonable for most people to take it supplementally on general principles, regardless of any particular therapeutic requirement.

Deficiencies of magnesium often occur in conjunction with a predisposing disease state such as chronic alcoholism, renal dysfunction, or following the use of certain medications. Hypertension, arrhythmias, neuromuscular manifestations, and personality changes are frequently the outcomes when a severe deficiency is present.

Certain diuretics, estrogen and oral contraceptives,

---

[18] In 1994 researchers at the Medical University in Charleston, South Carolina, undertook an investigation to determine if a relationship exists between low serum magnesium (Mg) levels and symptoms characteristic of peripheral neuropathy. After examining 68 patients they reported:

"Mg deficiency is a cause of sensory peripheral neuropathy-like symptoms in HIV disease. Mg replacement appears to be a beneficial treatment for sensory neuropathics [sic] in late stage HIV disease, both reducing morbidity and decreasing use of pain medications. Mg levels should be evaluated in HIV patients presenting with sensory neuropathy." *Int Conf AIDS* (1994 Aug 7–12; 10 (1): 202 abstract no. PB0235).

zinc, potassium and manganese all may increase magnesium requirements. It is also suggested that magnesium doses should be separated from taking the following medications by at least two hours: ACE inhibitors, antibiotics in the tetracycline or quinolone families (such as Cipro), Dilantin, Zantac, Pepid, and Macrodantin. (Magnesium is an active ingredient in antacids and laxatives.)

Kelp is very high in magnesium. Other excellent food sources are wheat bran, wheat germ, almonds, and cashews. Also appreciable quantities can be obtained from collard greens, avocado, sweet corn, cheddar cheese, and dried fruit.

This nutrient is considered quite safe taken in supplement form. Toxicity, when it occurs, is more often associated with kidney failure, when the kidney loses the ability to remove excess magnesium. The elderly are particularly at risk of magnesium toxicity because kidney function declines with age and older people are more likely to take magnesium-containing laxatives and antacids. Signs of excessive magnesium levels can be somewhat similar to magnesium deficiency and include mental status changes, nausea, diarrhea, appetite loss, muscle weakness, difficulty breathing, extremely low blood pressure, and irregular heartbeat.

Selenium

Selenium is a powerful **antioxidant**. Additionally it serves as a constituent of the enzyme **glutathione peroxidase**, which interacts with vitamin E in preventing free radicals from stealing electrons away from healthy cells. Selenium also reinforces the body's immune defenses. (People infected with the HIV virus frequently suffer from a selenium deficiency.) Moreover it has **anti-inflammatory** properties, reinforced when taken in conjunction with vitamin E and other vitamin antioxidants. A December 1998 study pointed out how **selenium** and **zinc** (as well as copper) fight free radicals together.[19]

Several studies have referred to an epidemic of optic and peripheral neuropathy that occurred in Cuba in the early 1990s. Patients who developed neuropathy during the epidemic were found to have had lower blood concentrations of riboflavin, vitamin E, **selenium**, alpha- and beta-carotenes, and the carotenoid lycopene. The inference drawn was that the neuropathies were associated

---

[19] *Clin Lab Med* (1998; 18 (4): 673–85):

"Copper, zinc, and selenium are involved in destruction of free radicals through cascading enzyme systems. Superoxide radicals are reduced to hydrogen peroxide by superoxide dismutases in the presence of copper and zinc cofactors. Hydrogen peroxide is then reduced to water by the selenium-glutathione peroxidase couple. Efficient removal of these superoxide free radicals maintains the integrity of membranes, reduces the risk of cancer, and slows the aging process. On the other hand, excess intake of these trace elements leads to disease and toxicity; therefore, a fine balance is essential for health. Trace element—deficient patients usually present with common symptoms such as malaise, loss of appetite, anemia, infection, skin lesions, and low-grade *neuropathy.*"

See also *Neurotoxicology* (1999 Dec; 20 (6): 935–44):

"The enzymes catalase and superoxide dismutase and the antioxidant agent *selenium* showed some protection against hydrazine neurotoxicity, suggesting an involvement of the generation of reactive oxygen species in the pathogenesis of isoniazid *neuropathy* [a neuropathy caused by a chemical used in treating tuberculosis]."

with an impairment of protective antioxidant pathways because of these deficiencies.[20]

Selenium is considered another of the "trace" minerals because it is needed only in minute amounts—micrograms rather than milligrams. (The RDI is 70 mcg.) For general health maintenance the editors of the *UC Berkeley Wellness Letter* in their April 1997 issue contended that most people get as much as they need from their regular diets and that a multi-vitamin/mineral pill containing selenium taken daily should be sufficient in any event. Some practitioners suggest, however, a daily intake of 200–400 mcg for therapeutic purposes and most would agree that if you are taking medications that reduce stomach acid, such as H2 blockers or proton pump inhibitors, you may need extra selenium regardless of the absence of a disease state.

Major dietary sources of selenium include fish, shellfish, red meat, grains (depending on soil content), eggs, garlic, and liver. However even a diet replete with these foods will not give a typical person (much less a PNer) an adequate intake if the soil in which they were grown is lacking in selenium.[21]

Deficiency symptoms include muscular weakness, growth disorders, and pancreatic problems while nausea,

---

[20] See, e.g., *American Journal of Clinical Nutrition* (2000 Jun; 71 (6 Suppl): 1676S-81S).

[21] To give an example of the effect of selenium soil depletion: China has very low rates of colon cancer, which is thought to be because of their people's typical low fat diet. However, in some parts of China where the soil is depleted of selenium, the incidence of various types of cancer is much higher than in the rest of the country.

abdominal pain and diarrhea, fatigue and irritability, are signs of toxicity which might occur at dosages in excess of 850 mcg on a daily basis.[22]

Zinc

Zinc functions in over 200 **enzymatic reactions** in the body and is involved in the synthesis and conversion of carbohydrates, lipids, and proteins to useable forms. It is also necessary for the production of brain **neurotransmitters**.

Deficiency of zinc is said to lead to impaired conduction and nerve damage. Dr. Robert Atkins of the Atkins Center for Complementary Medicine, claims that zinc deficiency is implicated in a whole range of neurological and neuropsychiatric disorders. He cites an investigation at the Department of Biochemistry, University of Missouri, which found that zinc deficiency in chicks and guinea pigs correlated with signs of peripheral neuropathy and that they were readily reversed by zinc therapy.[23]

A double-blind randomized study was conducted in India on 50 human subjects, including 20 healthy controls, 15 diabetic patients with neuropathy who received placebo for 6 weeks (Group—IIA), and 15 patients with diabetic neuropathy who were given supplemental zinc

---

[22] According to the *Merck Manual*, however, very high doses of this protective mineral can cause peripheral neuropathy (17th edition, 1999).

[23] *Journal of Nutrition* (2000; 130:1432S-36S).

sulphate (660 mg daily) for 6 weeks (Group-IIB). Serum zinc level, fasting blood sugar and post-prandial (after eating) blood sugar levels and motor nerve conduction velocity as markers were estimated on the first day and after 6 weeks in all subjects. At baseline (the beginning), serum zinc levels were significantly lower in group IIA and IIB as compared to the healthy controls. After 6 weeks the change in pre- and post- therapy markers were highly significant for group IIB along with insignificant changes in group IIA. No improvement in autonomic dysfunction was observed in either group. The investigators concluded, therefore, that oral zinc supplementation helps in achieving better glycemic control and in improvement in severity of peripheral neuropathy.[24]

The RDI for zinc is 15 mg. The mineral is considered toxic in large doses and can cause nausea and diarrhea. It also has been suggested that if any zinc supplementation is carried on over a long period of time copper supplementation should be undertaken as well since copper could be depleted in the body. (Steven Bratman, M.D., says the "with sufficiently excessive zinc intake, even taking extra copper won't help—the body will simply reject it.) Experts say that many multi-vitamin pills probably contain sufficient copper for this purpose.[25]

---

[24] *Assoc Physicians India* (Nov 1998; 46 (11): 939–42).

[25] A study measuring and comparing urinary excretions of manganese, chromium and copper among diabetics found that there was a "significantly higher urinary excretion" of copper by those who had diabetic neuropathy compared with diabetics who did not. *Diabetes Research* (1991 Nov; 18(3): 129–34.) This would suggest that PNers

Zinc is not often used in therapeutic dosages. Occasionally it is taken supplementally for the common cold in the form of lozenges containing 13 to 23 mg of zinc every two hours.

This mineral is widely distributed in foods. Red meat and poultry provide most of the zinc found in American diets. Other good food sources include beans, nuts, certain seafood, whole grains, fortified breakfast cereals, and dairy products. (Oysters contain more zinc by weight than any other food.)

Many general signs of zinc deficiency can appear, including growth retardation, hair loss, diarrhea, delayed sexual maturation and impotence, eye and skin lesions, and loss of appetite. There is also some evidence that weight loss, delayed healing of wounds, taste abnormalities, and mental lethargy can occur.

Lithium

In reviewing studies concerning mineral supplementation and its effects on peripheral neuropathy, I came across an interesting investigation in Japan in 2000 performed at the Osaka University Medical School. Clinicians tested the effects of **lithium** on the symptoms of rats that had been experimentally subjected to peripheral neuropathy. (Lithium, as you may know, is usually administered to counteract acute manic episodes in pa-

---

who decide to take supplemental zinc should be especially careful to make sure their tablets or capsules contain copper.

tients with bipolar affective disorders.[26] Also, maintenance therapy with the substance has been found useful
in preventing or diminishing the frequency of subsequent
relapses.)

The clinicians found PN symptoms reduced when they
used **intrathecal** injections (injections administered under the membranes covering the brain or spinal cord) of
lithium. Noting that this alkali metal already had found
widespread clinical application, they said their results
"suggested that its therapeutic utility may be extended to
include treatment of neuropathic pain symptoms resulting from peripheral nerve injury."[27]

Other studies I found where lithium was mentioned in
connection with peripheral neuropathy concerned its
toxic effects and its propensity to *induce* peripheral neuropathy. In one study two patients had developed acute

---

[26] An early paper entitled "A Review of Clinical Trials of Lithium in
Neurology," found that the mineral has been put to clinical trials in
no less than fifteen neurological disorders. They were Huntington's
chorea, tardive dyskinesia, spasmodic torticollis, Tourette's syndrome, L-dopa induced hyperkinesia and the "on-off" phenomenon in
Parkinsonism, organic brain disorders secondary to brain-injury,
drug induced delusional disorders, migraine and cluster headache,
periodic hypersomnolence, epilepsy, Meniere's disease and periodic
hypokalemic paralysis. The investigators found there were encour-
aging results on the use of lithium in cluster headaches, cyclic form
of migraine and hypomanic mood disorders due to organic brain disorders. *Pharmacol Biochem Behav* (1984; 21 Suppl 1: 57–64).

[27] *Pain* (2000 Mar; 85 (1–2): 59–64). In another study as reported in
Science News (November 11, 2000, Vol. 158, No. 20, 305–20), lithium
was found to have increased the volume of brain gray matter by about
3 percent in 8 of 10 people studied. The researchers proposed that
most of the increased volume resulted from nerve cells sprouting additional branches to nearby cells. They said that the use of the mineral should be studied in "various neurological disorders."

"sensorimotor polyneuropathy" after intoxication with lithium carbonate. Nerve conduction studies, electromyography, and sural nerve biopsy proved the syndrome to be an axonal neuropathy. Recovery of muscle strength, reflexes, and sensory function started weeks after discontinuation of lithium therapy. One patient fully recovered within a year. The investigators found nine other cases of lithium polyneuropathy in literature they surveyed.[28]

---

[28] *Muscle & Nerve* (1990 Mar; 13(3): 204–208). See also "Lithium and its Effects on the Endocrine System, Bones and Peripheral Nerves," *Fortschr Neurol Psychiatr* (1995 Apr; 63 (4): 149–61).

Chapter 4

Other Supplements

There are a number of other nutrient substances that can be considered for dealing with peripheral neuropathy which are not vitamins or minerals. They are discussed in this chapter.

Essential Fatty Acids

Essential fatty acids or EFAs are components of **cell membranes** the body needs but cannot manufacture itself. Diets rich in polyunsaturated fats such as EFAs increase the fluidity of these membranes. On the other hand diets high in saturated fats tend to lead to rigid and unhealthy cell membranes.[1]

EFAs are also precursors of **prostaglandins.** These substances are **hormones** that facilitate many processes such as energy production, the transfer of oxygen into the

---

[1] Saturated fatty acids are solid at room temperature—the greater the saturated fat content, the higher the melting temperature. Animal fats fall into this category. Polyunsaturated vegetable oils stay liquid at colder temperatures. The lower the temperature at which solidification occurs, the greater the degree of unsaturation.

bloodstream and the manufacture of hemoglobin. In addition to transporting oxygen, their particular importance to us lies in their assistance in the transmission of nerve impulses and possibly in the enhancement of nerve regeneration.

There are two main EFA groups: **omega-3** and **omega-6** fatty acids (technically both are **polyunsaturated** fatty acids). The terms refer to their differing chemical structures. Among the omega-3 acids are **eicosapentaenoic (EPA)** and **docosahexaenoic (DHA)** acids, which are found principally in **cold-water fish** such as sardines, herring, mackerel, salmon, and halibut. (Non-fish eaters can also try marine plants such as seaweed supplied as micro-algae supplements.)[2] Another omega-3, **alpha-linolenic acid**, is found mainly in flaxseed oil (a.k.a. linseed oil), canola oil, soybeans, and dark green leafy vegetables. The omega-3 **stearidonic acid** is found mainly in rarer types of seeds and nuts, including black currant seeds.

Omega-6s are principally found in many vegetable oils and plant products, one of the more important being **gamma-linolenic acid (GLA)**. Other omega-6s include **linoleic acid** (itself a precursor of GLA), and **arachidonic acid** (present in meat products).

Lowering the intake of sugar and alcohol in the diet may increase **EFA effectiveness**. Nutrients that as-

---

[2] Artemis Simopolous, M.D., head of the Center for Genetics, Nutrition and Health in Washington D.C., points out that another plant, purslane, is not only rich in omega-3s but also contains vitamins E and C as well as beta-carotene and glutathione—all valuable for PN-ers, as discussed in *Toes and Soles*. Purslane can be eaten cooked like spinach, or used fresh in salads.

sist EFA uptake are said to be the B-complex vitamins, vitamin C, magnesium, and zinc. As with any supplement, EFA effectiveness can be augmented with a nutritious, high fiber diet that emphasizes fresh and natural foods.

1. Omega-3s

There is a relative **deficiency** of omega-3 acids in most diets, a particularly troublesome fact for PNers. A paper in the *Journal of Nutrition* put it this way: "In humans with neuropathy or impairment of the immune system, significant deficits of omega-3 EFAs have been found."[3]

A study in the same journal, performed later in 1998 in Marseille, France, compared the feeding of olive oil and **fish oil** (a source of two omega-3 acids, as noted) to "small animal models" (whenever you see that phrase you can be pretty sure they mean rats) in which diabetic neuropathy had been induced. The investigators said their data suggested that fish oil therapy "may be effective in the *prevention* of diabetic neuropathy [my emphasis]."[4] Other French investigators the same year designed a test to determine the **protective effect** of a fish oil-rich diet on diabetic neuropathy. Diabetes was induced in laboratory rats who were then fed chow supplemented with either fish oil or olive oil. The investigators found a "significant beneficial effect on nerve conduction velocity," a marker

[3] 1998 Feb; 128 (2): 427S-433S.
[4] *Journal of Nutrition* (1999 Jan; 129 (1): 207–213).

in assessing neuropathy, with respect to the animals given the fish oil-fortified chow.[5]

Canadian doctors studied a 13-year-old boy with peripheral neuropathy. At 11 years of age, he was started on **cod liver oil** extract, high in DHA content. Over 12 months, he was reported to have demonstrated a marked clinical recovery. Nerve conduction studies showed reappearance of previously absent nerve responses and the amplitudes on motor nerve conduction velocities significantly increased. The improvements were said to have been from 7- to 14-fold.[6]

Investigators in this country studied a highly purified form of EPA (one of the omega-3 acids found in fish, as noted) that they labeled EPA-E. The substance was an "ethyl esterification" of natural EPA with a purity greater than 91%. The substance was administered orally to patients with diabetic neuropathies at a dose of 1800 mg/day for 48 weeks. At the end of the period they found that EPA-E had improved neuropathic symptoms in the lower extremities by about 50%. The investigators concluded that this highly purified form of EPA would have "significant beneficial effects on diabetic neuropathy."[7]

---

[5] *Journal of Neurochemistry* (1998 Aug; 71 (2): 732–40). We live in an imperfect world where clinical studies do not always provide consistent conclusions. A Scottish study of two-year old rats in which diabetic neuropathy had been induced and nerve conduction measurements made, found little neuropathic benefit from fish oil administration. *Diabetologia* (1993 Nov; 36 (11): 1132–38). Yet the preponderance of evidence seems to go the other way.

[6] *Neurology* (1999 Feb; 52(3): 640–43).

[7] *Journal of Diabetes and Its Complications* (1996; 10/5: 280–87).

An interesting study performed in Poland considered a different way to increase the intake of omega-3s without radical changes of eating patterns. The method involved the enrichment of regularly consumed foods with **un-hydrogenated** fish oil. The aim of the study was to establish sensory and nutritionally acceptable enrichment levels of low-calorie spreadable fats (soft margarine or a mix of butter and vegetable oil) with EPA and DHA by the addition of fish oil preparations. It was shown that spreadable fats might be enriched up to 1% EPA and DHA and that this had no significant influence on sensory acceptability.[8]

Another study, this one in Northern Ireland, was directed at the **bioavailability** of omega-3 fatty acids in foods enriched with **microencapsulated** fish oil. Twenty-five volunteers were randomly assigned to one of two groups for a 4-week intervention. One group received 0.9 g of omega-3 each day in a fish oil capsule (capsule group), while the second group (food group) received an equal amount from **enriched foods**. The investigators found no significant difference in the amount of arachidonic acid (another omega-3 fatty acid, as noted), EPAs, or DHAs, in blood platelets between the two groups following the intervention. They concluded omega-3s from microencapsulated fish-oil-enriched foods are as bioavailable as when supplemented by capsules. In their view "fortification of foods with microencapsulated fish oil of-

---

[8] *International Journal of Food Science Nutrition* (2001 Nov; 52 (6): 469–76).

fers an effective way of increasing [omega-3] intakes and status in line with current dietary recommendations."[9]

2. Omega-6s

Omega-6s are constituents of many vegetable oils such as **borage seed** and **black currant** as well as **evening primrose oil. Gamma linolenic acid (GLA)** is a specific and very important omega-6 fatty acid manufactured in the body by **linoleic acid**, which happens to be yet another omega-6. Various foods actually contain small amounts of GLA, and the body produces the fatty acid on its own from a number of dietary fats.

Evening primrose oil (EPO) offers a concentrated source of GLA, with 7 to 10% of its fatty acids available in that form. However, borage oil (BO) contains even more GLA (20 to 26%), and black currant oil (BC) offers 14 to 19%. The effectiveness and safety of the latter two have not been as intensively examined as for evening primrose oil. Nonetheless, some people prefer borage and black currant oils because they require a lower dose (at less total cost) for the same amount of GLA. Before you jump too fast, note should be made of a study reporting that even though the GLA concentration in BO is roughly twice as high as in primrose oil, **GLA-related effects**, such as the formation of **prostaglandins**, are comparable for both dietary oils on a per gram basis.[10] Also, where EPO

---

[9] *Annals of Nutrition & Metabolism* (2000; 44 (4): 157–62).
[10] *The Journal of Nutrition* (Sep 1998; 128 (9): 1411–14).

was pitted against BO and BC in a study involving the correction of motor and sensory nerve conduction velocity deficits in streptozotocin-diabetic rats, EPO "consistently outperformed" the other two.[11]

GLA has proven markedly helpful to people with neuropathy. In one investigation, 111 patients with mild diabetic neuropathy were randomized into a double-blind, placebo-controlled study at a dosage of 480 mg of GLA in the form of evening primrose oil daily. Various thresholds, sensations, tendon reflexes, and muscle strength were assessed by standard tests in upper and lower limbs. For the 16 parameters measured, changes over a one-year period in response to GLA were more favorable than any changes with placebo, and for 13 of these parameters, the difference was "statistically significant." The stated conclusion was that "GLA had a beneficial effect on the course of diabetic neuropathy."[12]

A recent study involving the use of GLA for diabetic neuropathy treatment in rats found that this omega-6 was helpful in preventing a deficit in nerve conduction velocity (NCV) which, as noted before, is a test and marker for peripheral neuropathy.[13] Also the June 2000 issue of the German journal, *Fortschritte der Neurologie-Psychiatrie,* reported that "evening primrose oil, containing gamma-

---

[11] *Prostaglandins Leukot Essential Fatty Acids* (1996 Sep; 55(3): 159–65).

[12] *Diabetes Care* (Jan 1993; 16(1): 8–15).

[13] *American Journal of Clinical Nutrition* (2000 Jan; 71(1 Suppl): 386S-92S). NCV, as mentioned before, is a measure of how fast electrical impulses flow through a nerve.

linolenic acid, might improve nerve conduction velocities, temperature perception, muscle strength, tendon reflexes, and sensory function."[14]

Another study I came across in an Internet "bio FAQ" format also suggested that patients with *existing* neuropathies could experience improvement with GLA supplementation. This study maintained that any one with diabetes might consider supplementing with borage oil— just mentioned as another omega 6 source—as a *preventive measure* against neuropathy. Two grams of borage oil daily was the recommended amount.[15] (Dr. Lark Lands, in her upcoming book, *Positively Well: Living with HIV as a Chronic, Manageable, Survivable Disease*, says that at least two borage oil capsules with 240 mg of GLA in each, taken on a daily basis, might be useful in dealing with neuropathy.)

One investigation noted the **synergistic effect** of combining GLA and alpha-lipoic acid in the treatment of diabetic neuropathy.[16] This work was affirmed in a later study reported in the same journal. The conclusion reached was that alpha-lipoic acid by itself did not improve nerve conduction velocity but a **conjugate** (a chemical compound formed by the union of compounds) of the two did.[17] Another study reported that GLA effects in dealing with peripheral neuropathy were "markedly enhanced" when given in combination with ascorbate (vita-

---

[14] *2000 Jun; 68 (6): 278–88.*

[15] *www.bioriginal.com.*

[16] *Diabetologia* (1998 April; 41 (4): 390–99).

[17] *Diabetologia* (1998 July; 41 (7): 839–43).

min C) as ascorbyl-GLA.[18] Yet another study noted the "marked synergistic interactions" between GLA and *antioxidants in general*.[19]

3. Getting the EFA Balance Right

It is said that people are more likely to consume too much of omega-6 fatty acids and too little of omega-3s. A few scientists claim that typical American diets contain 20 times as much omega-6s as omega-3s. Baruj Benacerraf, M.D., President Emeritus of the Dana-Farber Cancer Institute (a teaching affiliate of the Harvard Medical School) and recipient of the 1980 Nobel prize in medicine, goes further and says that people living in industrialized societies consume up to *30 times* more omega-6 than omega-3 fatty acids. He also says that omega-6 metabolic products (such as inflammatory prostaglandins; thromboxanes, which are active compounds that cause contraction of the arteries; and leukotrienes, which are active compounds that have potent actions on many organs and body systems) are sometimes produced in excessive amounts, causing allergic and inflammatory disorders and making the body more prone to heart attacks, strokes, and cancer.

---

[18] *Diabetes* (1997 Sep; 46 Suppl 2: S31–37). Another study in the same issue reported that "two multicenter, randomized, placebo-controlled trials in humans with diabetic neuropathy have shown significant benefits of GLA as compared with placebo in neurophysiological parameters, thermal thresholds, and clinical sensory evaluations." *Diabetes* (1997 Sep; 46 Suppl 2: S90–93).

[19] *Diabetes Research and Clinical Practice* (1999 Sep; 45 (2–3): 137–46).

Dr. Artemis Simopoulos points out that human beings in the beginning consumed a diet having approximately equal amounts of omega-3 and omega-6 fatty acids but that with the advent of vegetable oil consumption and greater meat intakes, the **balance** has **tipped** strongly to the latter.[20]

There are quite different ideas on an appropriate ratio of gamma-6s, and the products that contain them, to gamma-3s and their associated host products.[21] Many experts say, though, that a ratio of **three omega-6s to one omega-3s** is appropriate for most people.[22]

4. Therapeutic Dosages and Effects

Therapeutic dosages of omega-6s for diabetic neuropathy, based on GLA, are frequently in the 400 to 600 mg range. This is equivalent to about 4 to 6 grams of eve-

---

[20] *American Journal of Clinical Nutrition* (1999 Sept; 70 (3 Suppl): 560-S-569-S).

[21] "Scientists use the ratio of omega-6 fatty acids to omega-3 fatty acids to assess the balance between essential fatty acids in the diet. Research scientists from around the world recommend ratios varying from 5:1 to 10:1, while some experts suggest a ratio of between 1:1 and 4:1 as being optimal. The current ratio in our diet is estimated to be 14:1 to 20:1 with some studies indicating higher ratios in vegetarian populations compared to omnivorous populations." From "Essential Fatty Acids in Vegetarian Nutrition," by Brenda Davis, R. D.

[22] One expert says that although a ratio of 3 to 1 or 4 to 1 is well and good from a regular diet (he says that since the omega-3s are preferentially metabolized in the body, such ratios will assure a balanced composition at the cellular level), when you supplement with "longer chain derivatives" such as GLA and EPA/DHA (from fish oil, for example), a ratio of 1:1 would be more desirable (Barrie Carlsen, in the *Nutrition Digest*).

ning primrose oil or 2 to 3 grams of borage oil. Therapeutic dosages of fish oils (for the omega-3s) seem to run from 3 to 9 grams daily. In order to match the dosages used in several major studies you should probably take enough fish oil daily to supply about 1.8 grams (1800 mg) of EPA and .9 grams (900mg) of DHA. (Based on the amounts of those two EFAs in the fish oil soft gels I take that works out to 4–5 soft gels daily of 1000 mg strength since mine deliver only about 60% total EFAs. Others are available, though, that deliver 80% EFAs.) Incidentally, this requirement could also be covered by the weekly consumption of 2 to 3 portions of fatty fish.

Symptoms of EFA deficiencies or imbalances when they occur are said to include dry or scaly skin, excessively dry hair, fatigue, weakness, frequent infections, and mood disorders.

Harmful side effects with most EFA supplements are rare because EFAs are considered largely nontoxic. In fact over 4000 people have reportedly taken GLA or evening primrose oil in scientific studies with no adverse effects having been noted. However, cod liver and fish oil supplements can cause vitamin A and D toxicity when taken in excess. Effects of those toxicities include headaches, skin discoloration, fatigue, nausea, and gastrointestinal problems. (Fish oil supplements that have vitamins A and D removed are available.) Moreover, because fish oil has a mild blood-thinning effect it should not be combined with powerful blood-thinning medications such as Coumadin (warfarin) or heparin except on a physician's advice.

Alpha-Lipoic Acid

There are probably more studies attesting to the benefits of **alpha-lipoic acid (ALA),** also known as lipoic acid or thioctic acid, for dealing with peripheral neuropathy than studies for any other nutrient. ALA is a sulfur-containing fatty acid found inside every cell of the body, where it helps generate the energy that keeps us alive and functioning. This nutrient is a key part of the metabolic machinery that turns glucose (blood sugar) into energy for the body's needs.

Dr. Lester Packer, who heads the Department of Molecular & Cell Biology at the University of California, Berkley, calls ALA a **"universal antioxidant."** In addition to its remarkable abilities as a natural antioxidant, protecting nerves from oxidative damage and inflammation, it has great facility for raising levels of the enzyme **glutathione**, itself a powerful antioxidant.[23] Some research also suggests that the nutrient may be able to do the work of other antioxidants when the body is deficient in them. As a corollary, it has been demonstrated that ALA can regenerate other antioxidants such as vitamins A and C as well as coenzyme Q10.

ALA offers **dual antioxidant protection** because it

---

[23] Glutathione protects nerves and virtually all other tissues in the body from oxidative damage by free radicals. A study in the *Journal of Trace Elements* (2000; 13: 105–111), maintains that although dietary supplements of this enzyme are available, they are not well absorbed by the GI tract and are therefore ineffective. In the Journal article Dr. J. Aseth confirms that the antioxidant nutrients alpha-lipoic acid, vitamin C and vitamin E all help regenerate the body's glutathione.

is both fat and water soluble. Water solubility means that it works inside the nerve cell. Its fat solubility permits it to work outside the cell, at the membrane level. This double action on both sides of nerve cell walls is said to result in a stronger defense against damaging **free radicals**. (As mentioned before, we encounter these harmful molecular fragments every day through exposure to the sun's rays, automobile exhaust, smoke from various sources, and air pollution in general.)

The classic early study on the efficacy of alpha-lipoic acid for peripheral neuropathy, referred to as the **ALADIN study** (Alpha-Lipoic Acid in Diabetic Neuropathy), was performed in Dusseldorf, Germany, in 1995. The effects of ALA were studied in a 3-week multi-center, randomized, double-blind placebo-controlled trial, in 328 non-insulin-dependent diabetic patients with symptomatic peripheral neuropathy. These patients were randomly assigned to treatment with intravenous infusion of alpha-lipoic acid at three dose levels (1200, 600, or 100 mg), or placebo. Neuropathic symptoms (pain, burning, *paresthesia*, and numbness) were scored at baseline and at each visit. Based on the study results the investigators said that using intravenous treatment at a dose level of 600 mg daily was effective in reducing symptoms of peripheral neuropathy without causing significant adverse reactions.[24]

Clinical evidence from various parts of the world continues to support the use of ALA for diabetic and other peripheral neuropathies. A randomized, double-blind

---

[24] *Diabetologia* (1995 Dec; 38 (12): 1425–33).

study at the University of Zagreb in Croatia in 1999, concluded that after the daily administration of 600 mg of ALA to one group of diabetic patients and 1200 mg to another for a period of two years (65 patients in all), ALA "appeared to have a beneficial effect on several attributes of nerve conduction."[25] (The investigators did qualify their opinion by saying that although neuropathic symptoms seemed to have improved over the 24 month study period, the "long-term response remains to be established.")

A three-week study performed in Dusseldorf, Germany, reached a similar conclusion. The patients with diabetic neuropathy enrolled there were given 600 mg of ALA three times daily. Researchers made the point that not only were neuropathy pain symptoms lessened but the nutrient was well tolerated.[26]

Russian investigators also found symptomatic improvement in a group of 29 patients with diabetic neuropathy after 14 days of ALA.[27]

Similarly, American investigators at the Mayo Clinic in Rochester, Minnesota, found that after the adminis-

---

[25] *Free Radical Research* (1999 Sep; 31(3): 171–79).

As previously noted, results from clinical studies sometimes are measured in terms of objective parameters such as vibration threshold and nerve conduction velocity.

[26] *Diabetic Medicine* (1999 Dec; 16(12): 1040–43). To give perspective, I should report that another German study came to a different conclusion, finding "no effect on neuropathic symptoms distinguishable from placebo." They admitted, though, that their findings might have been off the mark because the various centers where the 509 patients in the study were examined were using different scoring methods [tsch!] (*Diabetes Care*, 1999 Aug; 22 (8): 1296–1301). Interestingly, two of the investigators in this study were investigators in both the Zagreb and Dusseldorf studies just mentioned!

[27] *Zb Nevrol Psikhiatr Im S S Korsakova* (1999; 99(6): 18–22).

tration of ALA, peripheral nerve function improved in rats in which diabetic neuropathy had previously been induced.[28]

A more recent study delved into the nitty-gritty of the *way* ALA offers antioxidant protection.[29] Researchers in Germany investigated the effects of the nutrient on the body's **microcirculation system** for carrying oxygen to nerve cells. (This system consists of blood vessels such as capillaries with a diameter of less than 300 micrometers. Peripheral neuropathy is sometimes associated with a lack of blood circulation to the nerve cells.) The investigators concluded that microcirculation was benefited by the administration of either 600 mg or 1200 mg daily over a six-week period. In technical terms they found that there was a decrease in the "time to peak capillary blood cell velocity,"—a marker in determining oxygen transport benefit.[30]

---

[28] *Diabetes* (1999 Oct; 48 (10): 2045–51). Apparently, though, not all rats are the same. A study in the Netherlands found only minor beneficial effects from alpha-lipoic acid and that these effects were insufficient to improve nerve conduction deficits in their diabetic rats. *European Journal of Clinical Investigation* (2001 May; 31 (5): 417–24). Perhaps there *is* something different about rats bred in the Netherlands. Another study from that country in 2001 found that a conjugate of GLA and ALA failed to reverse *established* deficits in nerve conduction velocity in their rats induced with diabetic neuropathy; the investigators acknowledged that there was a body of evidence establishing that GLA-ALA *did* improve *early* deficits in such conduction. *Journal of the Neurological Sciences* (2001 Jan 1; 182 (2): 99–106).

[29] *Experimental and Clinical Endocrinology and Diabetes* (2000; 108 (3): 168–74).

[30] *Free Radical Research* (1999 Nov; 27 (9–10): 1114–20). Another study at the University of Michigan, reported in *Diabetes* (2000 Jun; 49(6): 1006–15), noted the "complex interrelationships among nerve

A study performed at the University of Texas South-western Medical Center at Dallas also examined the manner in which ALA functions as an antioxidant, concluding it does so because "it decreases plasma- and LDL-oxidation."[31]

Finally a meta analysis in Germany (which pre-dated the Texas study) examined the results of 15 clinical trials.[32] The conclusion, based on all 15, was that short-term (three weeks) treatment of diabetic neuropathy, using 600 mg per day of ALA, "appeared to reduce the chief symptoms" of neuropathy. Moreover, the preliminary data indicated to the investigators the "possible long-term im-

---

perfusion, energy metabolism, osmolyte content, conduction velocity, and oxidative stress that may reflect the heterogeneous and compartmentalized composition of peripheral nerve." In particular the researchers said the studies implicated *oxidative stress* as an important factor in diabetic neuropathy.

One study, in concluding alpha-lipoic therapy "improves and may prevent diabetic neuropathy," indicated that "oxidative stress appears to be primarily due to the processes of nerve ischemia [reduced blood flow] and hyperglycemia autooxidation." *In Vivo* (2000 Mar-Apr; 14 (2): 327–30). An interesting paper concerning impaired blood flow with restricted oxygen delivery to peripheral nerves, implicates the accumulation of heavily glycated proteins within the arterial walls, resulting in "chronic vasoconstriction." *Free Radical Biology and Medicine* (2000 Feb 15; 28 (4): 652–56).

[31] *Free Radical Biology and Medicine* (1999 Nov; 27 (9–10): 1114–21).

A Russian study determined that alpha-lipoic acid also had a therapeutic effect in the nitric oxide and stress protein systems in diabetic patients with polyneuropathy. *Bulletin of Experimental Biology & Medicine* (2000 Oct; 130 (10): 986–90).

[32] In a meta analysis or study, the results from a number of selected trials are combined in order to come to general conclusions. It is often used when a number of small trials give conflicting or statistically insignificant results.

provement in motor and sensory nerve conduction in the lower limbs." The investigators emphasized that these 15 trials revealed a "highly favorable safety profile" for ALA.[33]

A more recent paper, also from Germany and mentioned in the discussion of GLA, again acknowledged the benefits of ALA for the treatment of diabetic neuropathy: "Symptomatic therapy includes alpha-lipoic acid treatment, as the antioxidant seems to improve neuropathic symptoms."[34] (It should be noted that ALA is specifically approved for the treatment of diabetic neuropathy in Germany.)

Incidentally, in addition to painful sensory neuropathies, alpha-lipoic acid is useful with **autonomic neuropathies**. These disorders, which affect involuntary or semi-voluntary functions such as control of inner organs, are common among people with diabetes and have been reported to be present in up to 40% of Type 2 diabetic patients. Symptoms may include gastroparesis (a condition where the stomach is not emptying properly and characterized by nausea, vomiting, and abdominal distension), sexual dysfunction, low blood pressure when standing up (postural hypotension), and inability to sweat, as well as a variety of cardiac abnormalities.

An earlier German study showed that alpha-lipoic acid caused a significant improvement in irregular heart rate

---

[33] *Experimental and Clinical Endocrinology and Diabetes* (1999; 107 (7): 421–30).

[34] *Fortschritte der Neurologie-Psychiatrie* (2000 Jun; 68 (6): 278–88).

in subjects with autonomic neuropathy.[35] (Richard N. Podell, M.D., who has studied ALA extensively, maintains that this study "provides the first clear evidence that nutritional treatment alone can reverse the course of autonomic neuropathy.")

There is no daily requirement established for ALA, presumably because a healthy body makes enough of it to supply daily energy requirements. However some practitioners recommend supplementation regularly because of its superior antioxidant capabilities; Lester Packer, Ph. D., considered an expert in this area, recommends daily dietary additions of 100 mg.

Many health care professionals recommend dosage levels of 400–600 mg of ALA daily for **therapeutic** purposes. In fact some go as high as 1200 mg per day. There reportedly have been no serious adverse effects from the use of ALA, even in quite high dosages (up to 1800 mg daily). Minor effects have been mainly allergic skin reactions.

If you are looking for natural sources of this nutrient, liver and yeast contain small amounts.

Acetyl-L-Carnitine

This is an **amino acid** normally not considered an "essential" nutrient because the body can manufacture whatever most people need. However, supplemental ALC (which is the acetyl ester and more bioavailable form of carnitine) may improve the ability of certain tissues to produce energy.

---

[35] *Diabetes Care* (1997; 20: 369–73).

ALC is vital in the transport of fats into mitochondria (the powerhouses of the cells) and assists in the production of acetylcholine—one of the body's key neurotransmitters.

The claimed benefits of **acetyl-l-carnitine** for us are said to be based on the nutrient's **neuroprotective** and **neuroenhancing** properties. The rationale is that ALC raises **myoinositol** content in the nerves.[36] (Myoinositol is the active form of **inositol,** as previously noted, the latter being a naturally occurring substance in the body which aids in the breakdown of fats.) Additionally, ALC is considered a good **antioxidant**.

There seems to be some diversity of opinion now, though, as to how useful ALC is for someone with PN (the same doubts as were raised with myoinositol, as you may recall from that discussion). Early studies were positive. For example investigators in Milan, Italy, working with diabetic animals, concluded in 1992 that ALC was potentially helpful in treating **autonomic neuropathies**.[37]

In a small double-blind study involving humans in Italy using intramuscular administrations of ALC, the nutrient was said to have resulted in "highly significant im-

---

[36] See, e.g., *J Pharmacol Exp Ther* (1998 Dec; 287 (3): 897–902): "ALC also increased the myo-inositol as well as the free-carnitine content without affecting the sorbitol content. These observations suggest that there is a close relationship between increased polyol pathway activity and carnitine deficiency in the development of diabetic neuropathy and that an aldose reductase inhibitor, TAT, and a carnitine alog, ALC, can have therapeutic potential for the treatment of diabetic neuropathy."

[37] *International Journal of Clinical Pharmacology Research* (1992; 12 (6): 225–30).

provement" in painful neuropathies. The antioxidant function of ALC was believed to have been the likely mechanism of action.[38]

That same year other investigators at the University of Chieti in Italy, reported that 31 patients injected with one gram of ALC daily for 15 consecutive days, experienced reduced pain from diabetic neuropathy.[39]

The following year another group of researchers from Milan were less enthusiastic, concluding that ALC probably represented "only a co-factor" in the "clinical picture of human diabetic neuropathy."[40] (Rats did better than humans that year; a Michigan study showed that ALC treatments promoted two-fold as much nerve fiber regeneration as in their untreated littermates.[41])

In 1997 investigators at the Catholic University Medi-

---

[38] *Diabetalogica* (1995; 38: 123).

[39] *International Journal of Clinical Pharmacology Research* (1995; 15 (1): 9–15).

[40] *Journal of the Peripheral Nervous System* (1996; 1(2): 157–63). This (mostly) same group of investigators seemed to reverse themselves the following year, at least with respect to one sub-population of people with PN. They there concluded, after studying ten patients with HIV-induced peripheral neuropathy who were treated with .5 to 1 gram of ALC for three weeks, that "acetyl-L-carnitine can have a role in the treatment of pain in distal polyneuropathy related to HIV infection." The investigators cautioned, however, that "further double-blind, placebo-controlled studies" were required to confirm their results. *Journal of the Peripheral Nervous System* (1997; 2 (3): 250–52).

[41] *Journal of Clinical Investigations* (1996 Apr 15; 97(8): 1900–07). Investigators in an Illinois study reported the following year that "ALC at a dose of 150 mg/Kg/d given for one month to streptozotocin-induced diabetic rats, produced near normalization of nerve conduction velocity with no adverse effects on glucose, insulin or free fatty acid levels." *Endocrinology Research* (1997 Feb-May; 23 (1–2): 27–36).

cal School in Rome considered "motornuclear changes after cranial nerve injury." They severed nerves in a number of animal models and then administered ALC at the site of injury to observe motor nerve regeneration. They found that the substance showed "significant neuroprotective effects," with positive implications for patients with a loss of nerve function.[42]

However, another contingent of Italian investigators again threw a blanket of doubt over the benefits of ALC in 1998. Referring to the famous Diabetes Control and Complications Trial (DCCT) and the so-called Stockholm studies, they acknowledged that careful maintenance of near-normal blood glucose levels was the best approach to "primary and secondary prevention of peripheral neuropathy." ALC, aldose-reductase inhibitors (discussed in *Toes and Soles* and *Toes and Woes*), gamma-linolenic acid, and antioxidants as a class, were all considered of "poor efficacy and often with significant adverse effects," in their rather gloomy view.[43]

The Japanese and the English appear to be in the opposite camp, investigators in those two countries both finding at least some merit in the use of ALC for treating peripheral neuropathy. The Japanese compared the effects of ALC and an aldose reductase inhibitor (known by its acronym, TAT, and referred to in a preceding footnote) on neural functions in rats where diabetic neuropathy had been induced. They concluded that both substances

---

[42] *Archives Italiennes de Biologie* (1997 Sep; 135(4): 343–51).
[43] *Drugs* (1997 Sep; 54(3): 414–21).

had "therapeutic potential for the treatment of diabetic neuropathy."[44]

In a paper presented in *Drug Safety*, two English clinicians reviewed the techniques for management of peripheral neuropathy in people with HIV infections. In their view, ALC and **nerve growth factors** such as recombinant human nerve growth factor (also discussed in my other two neuropathy books) are "agents that can helpfully assist" in managing PN.[45]

If you weigh it all out, the preponderance of evidence from these studies seems to be slightly in ALC's favor for treating PN.

Carnitine is found mainly in meat and dairy products. There is no dietary requirement for this nutrient. Some people are said to have a genetic defect that hinders their ability to make carnitine. In addition, diseases of the liver, kidneys, or brain may inhibit carnitine production.

Certain medications, especially the anti-seizure drugs valproic acid (Depakene) and phenytoin (Dilantin), may reduce carnitine levels; however, whether taking extra carnitine would be helpful in these cases has not been determined. Heart muscle tissue, because of its high-energy requirements, is particularly vulnerable to carnitine deficiency.

Typical therapeutic dosages of ALC range from 500 to 1,000 mg three times daily, and the substance appears to

---

[44] *Journal of Pharmacological Experimental Therapy* (1998 Dec; 287 (3): 897–902).
[45] *Drug Safety* (1998 Dec; 19 (6): 481–94).

be quite safe. However, individuals with low or border-line-low **thyroid levels** are warned to stay clear of carnitine because it might impair the action of thyroid hormones. Other possible side effects include occasional diarrhea, skin rash, and nausea. Individuals on dialysis should not take ALC without a physician's supervision.

Miscellaneous Supplements

In *Toes and Soles* and *Toes and Woes* just about every alternative treatment I came across that had any reasonable chance of success in dealing with our affliction was at least mentioned. The idea was that even if scientific evidence of efficacy for a particular treatment was somewhat lacking, it was discussed if it offered at least a *prospect* of working.

Based on that criterion, amino acids and metabolites such as N-acetyl cysteine (NAC), glutamine, coenzyme Q10 (CoQ10), S-adenosylmethione (SAMe), and methyl sulfonyl methane (MSM) were included even though in most instances there was only light scientific or anecdotal support for PN use. The same was true for a number of herbs discussed: St. John's wort, bioflavonoids, grape seed extract, and the following which were very briefly noted: cat's claw, feverfew, ginseng, green tea, hops flower, the Noni plant, and valerian root.

The purpose of this book is different, though, and a different inclusionary standard is being used. Here discussion is limited to supplements for which there is **credible**

scientific support for their employment.[46] Consequently, unless I found clinical studies to uphold their use, directly or inferentially (sorry if they weren't always peer reviewed, random, double-blinded, placebo controlled), they are not addressed. Since the ones listed in the preceding paragraph do not pass muster on that basis they are not being further considered. (This is not to say they should *never* be thought of, and maybe clinical work in the future will demonstrate more specific reasons for using some of them with greater confidence of benefit.)

Having said all of that, there are three rather off-the-beaten-path herbal substances that look increasingly intriguing for PNers and that bear mentioning here, based on clinical studies. The first is relatively well known, certainly to most regular supplement users. The next two are a little more (nay, a lot more) obscure. I have a hunch that may change in the next few years as more literature is developed concerning their uses.

1. Ginkgo Biloba

This is an extract made from leaves of the tree bearing the same name. The tree, also called the **maidenhair tree**, belongs to a species at least 300 million years old. The

---

[46] We need to have a sound basis for spending our money on nutrient supplements. Let's not willy-nilly accept some of the mysterious formulations being sold for PN such as the following: "a proprietary blend of albumin, essential oils, oriental herbs, enzymatically predigested botanical extracts, mineral and vitamin complexes, antioxidants and glucosamine." I challenge anybody to tell me exactly what you would be getting that would help you (as well as what side effects you might be risking)!

extract is said to be the most widely prescribed herb in Germany and the scientific record for its use is extensive.

Ginkgo biloba's principal therapeutic value arises from its **antioxidant properties**. There is also evidence that it helps in cases of impaired mental performance and enhances short-term memory by regulating **neurotransmission**. In fact the extract has been shown to be effective in both the prevention and early intervention of **CNS disorders** associated with aging. In this respect it appears to act by facilitating improved blood flow through the body and especially through the brain.

There reportedly have been more than 50 double-blind clinical studies performed in Europe showing its favorable effects on both vascular insufficiency and age-related decreases in brain function.

A 1993 study examined the neuropathic efficacy of a component of ginkgo biloba in small mammals. In an experimental model designed to mimic peripheral neuropathy based on traumatic damage to sciatic nerves, results showed improved **functional nerve regeneration**.[47]

An analysis of 15 European studies on the herb was reported in an *Archives of Family Medicine* article, "A Review of 12 Commonly Used Medicinal Herbs."[48] The report indicated ginkgo biloba caused an overall reduction in claudication (lameness or limping) symptoms of the subjects examined and permitted a 50% increase in their pain-free walking. (Although many PNers certainly can relate to the walking part it wasn't clear from the article

---

[47] *Planta Med* (1993 Aug; 59(4): 302–307).
[48] 1998 Nov-Dec; 7 (6): 523–36.

whether the problems experienced by the subjects had been circulatory or neurological.)

In 1999 Japanese investigators reviewed a number of studies concerning the ginkgo biloba extract, GBLE. They reported that:

> [The extract] has an antioxidant action as a free radical scavenger, a relaxing effect on vascular walls, an antagonistic action on platelet-activating factor, an improving effect on blood flow or microcirculation, and a stimulating effect on inflammatory cells by suppressing the production of active oxygen and nitrogen species. GBLE inhibited the increase in the products of the oxidative decomposition low-density lipoprotein (LDL), reduced the cell death in various types of neuropathy, and prevented the oxidative damage to mitochondria, suggesting that GBLE exhibits beneficial effects on neuron degenerative diseases by preventing chronic oxidative damage.[49]

Some practitioners suggest taking 120 to 240 mg daily for therapeutic purposes. The authors of the *Archives of Family Medicine* article referred to above, however, would limit intake to 120 mg per day of standardized ginkgo (designated Egb 761).

Ginkgo has in the past been considered quite safe. However it has been linked to stroke in a very few cases, and there has been recent concern as to possible internal bleeding following use, particularly where blood-thinning drugs such as Coumadin (warfarin), heparin, or even aspirin or high-dose vitamin E, are being used. Laurence Kinsella, M.D., as mentioned before an expert on

---

[49] *Antioxidants & Redox Signalling* (1999 Winter; 1(4): 469–80).

nutrients and peripheral neuropathy, points out in this regard that this herb has caused intracranial hemorrhaging in some patients.

2. Goshajinkigan

Since the 4th century A.D. the Japanese have practiced a form of herbal medicine called "**kampo**." While Western herbal preparations are typically composed of a single herb, kampo formulations are generally **combinations** of four or more **botanical products**. The types and quantities in a given formulation are said to have been determined by experience through the centuries and are specified in classical medical texts.

The production of kampo extracts is regulated by the Drug Good Manufacturing Practices [Act] established by the Japanese Ministry of Health and Welfare (which incidentally insures greater adherence to strict quality control than obtains under unregulated manufacturing practices in this country[50]).

---

[50] The following from an "Overview of Dietary Supplements" (Food and Drug Administration, Center for Food Safety and Applied Nutrition, January 3, 2001), states the U.S. position:

"Manufacturers do not need to register themselves nor their dietary supplement products with FDA before producing or selling them. Currently, there are no FDA regulations that are specific to dietary supplements that establish a minimum standard of practice for manufacturing dietary supplements. However, FDA intends to issue regulations on good manufacturing practices that will focus on practices that ensure the identity, purity, quality, strength and composition of dietary supplements. At present, the manufacturer is responsible for establishing its own manufacturing practice guidelines to ensure that the dietary supplements it produces are safe and contain the ingredients listed on the label."

Most kampo formulations are taken in the form of prescriptions rather than as OTC medicines. One hundred and forty eight of these formulations are covered by Japan's national health insurance program. The herbal formulation **goshajinkigan (GJK),** which consists of 10 different herbs, is one of these.

Clinicians in New Zealand investigated the effects of this formulation on rats with streptozocin-induced diabetic neuropathy in 1995. They administered GJK by injection and after one week began a series of oral administrations. According to the investigators, nerve conduction velocity (as previously noted, a marker of neuropathy) had "improved significantly" by the end of the 16-week study period when compared to non-treated diabetic rats, although the treated rats were still not completely normalized. The investigators made the point that herbal medicines such as GJK, which is a combination of herbs, have "unique synergistic and synthetic effects that result from interactions between individual herbal components, and may induce a wide range of therapeutic potential and utility."[51]

In a study at the University of Yamanashi Medical School in 1994 involving 13 patients with diabetic neuropathy, the researchers concluded that the administration of 7.5 grams daily of goshajinkigan for three months relieved subjective symptoms and improved sensations in 9 of the 13.[52]

The information on this herbal substance is presented

---

[51] *Journal of Neurological Sciences* (1995 Oct; 132 (2): 177–81).
[52] *Diabetes Research and Clinical Practice* (1994; 26(2): 121–28).

only as a matter of possible interest to you; it is perhaps something to keep your eye on for future developments and availability.[53] But if you have a yen (or however many yen it takes—you might even have to go to Japan to buy it [54]) and want to try goshajinkigan now, let me not raise doubts in your mind by pointing out the name sounds a little like "gosh 'am jinxed agin."

3. Sangre de Grado

This remarkable substance was originally discussed in *Toes and Soles*. I have come across a new study which further establishes its treatment credibility for dealing with neuropathic problems.

Sangre de grado, or blood of the dragon, was the name given to the blood-red sap produced from a fast growing Amazonian tree by Spanish explorers. Indians living in the Amazon River basin had used it as an herbal remedy for hundreds of years before the time of the conquistadors. It is still widely sold in Peru for diarrhea, gastrointestinal discomfort, and ulcers.

In fact, clinical studies show that the sap has a number of uses both topically and internally. It performs, for example, as an **analgesic**, quieting the firing of pain signals to the brain from sensory nerve fibers.

In a clinical trial in Louisiana (as reported in *Natural*

---

[53] Laurence J. Kinsella, M.D., cautions that Chinese herbal remedies are sometimes laced with variable amounts of mercury, lead and arsenic, and can be neurotoxic.
[54] You could possibly find it in this country, however, in stores that cater to Japanese customers.

Science, May 15, 2000), pest control workers were said to have found relief from a variety of insect bites and stings within 90 seconds. The investigators found that sangre de grado offered pain relief and alleviated itching and swelling symptoms for up to six hours.

A study performed at the University of Antwerp in Belgium found that the sap stimulated wound contraction and helped in forming new collagen and regenerating skin. [55]

Still another study performed at the Department of Pediatrics and Center for Cardiovascular Sciences at the Albany Medical College, New York, concluded that sangre de grado is a "potent, cost-effective treatment for gastrointestinal ulcers and distress via anti-microbial, anti-inflammatory, and sensory afferent-dependent actions."[56]

A newer study performed at the same institution by essentially the same clinicians, investigated the use of a sangre de grado **balm** and concluded the substance is "a potent inhibitor of sensory afferent nerve mechanisms and [the investigators would] support its ethnomedical use for disorders characterized by neurogenic inflammation."[57]

The possible benefits of sangre de grado to PNers, according to Dr. John Wallace of the University of Calgary, are based on the facts that "it not only prevents pain sensations, it also blocks the tissue response to a chemical released by nerves that promotes inflammation." Wallace

---

[55] *Journal of Natural Products* (1993 Jun; 5 (6): 899–906).
[56] *American Journal of Physiology. Gastrointestinal and Liver Physiology* (2000 Jul; 279 (1): G192–200).
[57] *The Journal of Investigative Dermatology* (2001 Sep; 117 (3): 725–30).

claims there is no other substance which shares these two ends. He is so enthralled with the therapeutic prospects of this herb that he thinks "every medicine cabinet and first aid kit in North America will one day be stocked with medicines containing the sap."

Chapter 5

Practical Considerations

Following are a few general observations on matters mentioned in previous chapters. Also I have included my own thoughts, based on the evidence as I see it, for a sensible program of nutrient supplementation.

Bioavailability

The concept of **bioavailability** was referred to in connection with a few of the supplements discussed in this book. It has to do with the body's ability to **absorb** and **effectively utilize** the nutrients supplied to it orally or in some other manner. Specifically, it concerns how easily and completely supplements dissolve in the digestive tract and are then taken up by the blood cells for delivery to tissues where needed.[1]

---

[1] "Digestion refers to the chemical and physical modifications which render ingested food constituents absorbable by the small intestine. Absorption is the process by which the products of digestion pass through the digestive tract into the cells lining it, and from there into

The degree of bioavailability ultimately depends on several factors, including how long the nutrient remains in the gastrointestinal tract, what else a person is consuming at the time,[2] and his or her overall nutritional status. Also, as will be discussed, both the physical and the chemical forms of the nutrients taken are of importance.[3]

To be bioavailable supplements first must be supplied to the body in an **absorbable** form. (Whether the supplements are actually used or metabolized may be another matter.[4]) Orally administered nutrient supplements are absorbed from the gastrointestinal tract with absorption mostly taking place in the small intestine.[5] To reach the

---

the bloodstream or lymph." Ball, *Bioavailability and Analysis of Vitamins in Foods*, 6.

[2] Just to give one example: fiber can entrap nutrients, reducing the ability of the intestine to absorb them.

[3] Predicting bioavailability can be a bit tricky. As one clinician wrote:

> "Does the size of a nutrient dose matter? Does diet composition or meal frequency matter? Does the food matrix in which the nutrient is bound materially affect the nutrient's bioavailability? And if so, as seems likely, what happens if the food is puréed, juiced, cooked, or both cooked and mashed? This bioavailability problem seems to leave us with endless unanswered questions and a tremendous amount of work to do. However, bioavailability of specific nutrients is a cornerstone to determining the amount of any given nutrient for optimal health." *American Journal of Clinical Nutrition* (May 2000; 71 (5): 1029–1030).

[4] In a paper, "Factors in Aging that Affect the Bioavailability of Nutrients," Robert M. Russell makes the point that elderly people seem to have a higher need for vitamin B6, not because of a malabsorption problem but because of a problem in metabolism after absorption has occurred. *Journal of Nutrition* (Apr 2000; 131; (45): 1359S-61S).

[5] *Malabsorption* disorders—where nutrients aren't being absorbed properly into the bloodstream from the small intestine—may be caused by a broad spectrum of diseases. Diarrhea, bloating or cramping, frequent bulky stools, muscle wasting, and a distended abdomen

blood stream the supplement must pass through first the intestinal wall and then the liver. The intestinal wall and liver chemically alter many nutrients, decreasing the amount absorbed. In contrast, if the nutrients are injected intravenously they reach the blood stream without passing through the intestinal wall and liver, resulting in a shorter absorption process.

1. Physical Forms and Bioavailability

When being manufactured, a supplement is usually combined with other ingredients. Tablets, for example, are a mixture of nutrients and additives that function as disintegrants, stabilizers, and dilutents. The type and amount of additives and the degree of compression to form the pills affect how quickly the tablet dissolves. Drug manufacturers adjust these variables to optimize the rate and extent of the drug's absorption. The following explanation is from Chapter 6, Section 2, of the 17th edition of *The Merck Manual*. Although the discussion is directed to drugs, the process applies to nutrient supplements as well:

> If a tablet dissolves and releases the drug too quickly, it may produce a blood level of the active drug that provokes an excessive response. On the other hand, if the tablet doesn't dissolve and release the drug quickly

---

may accompany malabsorption.

    A nutrient may be *properly* absorbed and enter the circulation but may not be taken up by the tissues because they have reached saturation. In this case the excess nutrients may simply be excreted. Ball, *Bioavailability and Analysis*, 25.

enough, much of the drug may pass into the feces without being absorbed. Laxatives and diarrhea, which speed up passage through the gastrointestinal tract, may reduce drug absorption. Therefore, food, other drugs, and gastrointestinal diseases can influence drug bioavailability.

Consistency of bioavailability among drug products is desirable. Drug products that are chemically equivalent contain the same active drug but may have different inactive ingredients that can affect the rate and extent of absorption. The drug's effects, even at the same dose, may not be the same from one drug product to another. Drug products are bioequivalent when they not only contain the same active ingredient but also produce virtually the same blood levels over time. Bioequivalence thereby ensures therapeutic equivalence, and bioequivalent products are interchangeable.

Some drug products are specially formulated to release their active ingredients slowly—usually over 12 hours or more. These controlled-release dosage forms slow or delay the rate at which a drug is dissolved. For example, drug particles in a capsule may be coated with a polymer (a chemical substance) of varying thicknesses designed to dissolve at different times in the gastrointestinal tract.

Some tablets and capsules have protective (enteric) coatings that are intended to prevent irritants, such as aspirin, from harming the stomach lining or from decomposing in the acidic environment of the stomach. These dosage forms are coated with a material that doesn't begin to dissolve until it comes in contact with the less acidic environment or digestive enzymes of the small intestine. Such protective coatings don't always dissolve properly though, and many people, especially the elderly, pass such products intact in their feces.

Many other properties of solid dosage forms (tablets or capsules) affect absorption after oral administration. Capsules consist of drugs and other substances within a gelatin shell.[6] The gelatin swells and releases its contents when it becomes wet. The shell usually erodes quickly. The size of the drug particles and other substances affects how fast the drug dissolves and is absorbed. Drugs from capsules filled with liquids tend to be absorbed more quickly than those from capsules filled with solids.

A side note to the Merck explanation: the *U.S. Pharmacopeia*[7] sets standards for disintegration. According to these standards, disintegration for vitamin and mineral compounds should take place within about 35 minutes within the intestine. But that doesn't always happen. Undigested vitamin and mineral pills, in fact, present major problems for sewer systems. For example it is reported that 165 thousand pounds of such pills are pulled out of sewers in Tacoma, Washington, each month![8]

---

[6] It should be noted that pressed tablets would usually contain more nutrients than the equivalent size of capsules or soft gels.

[7] USP has a long history of setting standards for dietary supplements, dating back to the first *United States Pharmacopeia* published in 1820 that included only natural medicines. USP is now recognized in the Dietary Supplement Health and Education Act (DSHEA) amendments to the Federal Food, Drug and Cosmetic Act, as the nation's official compendia for dietary supplement standards.

[8] The *Physician's Desk Reference* (p.1542), maintains only about 10 to 20% of pills are absorbed. That compares with an absorption rate of 98% for liquid or spray forms of nutrient administration, according to the PDR. (I must say these numbers are hard to believe.) The ex-

2. Chemical Forms and Bioavailability

Studies have shown that, as mentioned in connection with several nutrients discussed earlier, some particular molecular forms are more **bioavailable** than others. The following is for those who might wish to delve into these "chemical connections" a little further. (Only those where the particular chemical form might make a difference to PNers are covered here.)

(a) Vitamin B1

As previously noted, the lipid or fat—soluble forms of thiamin or **vitamin B1—benfotiamine** and **allithiamine**—have greater bioavailabilty than water-soluble **thiamin hydrochloride** or **thiamin nitrate**. This is largely due to the fact that the thiamin in these fat-soluble types is stored and available in the body for a longer period than is true with respect to the water-soluble forms; in the latter instance the thiamin might very well be uselessly excreted before full benefits can be realized. Moreover, the fat-solubility of benfotiamine and allithiamine is said to permit superior penetration of cell membranes by the thiamin.

Incidentally G.F.M Ball, in *Bioavailability and Analysis of Vitamins* (p. 286), previously referred to, notes an

---

planation is that liquid forms bypass the digestive process and go directly into the blood stream and into cells within a matter of minutes, somewhat similar to intravenous injection. All of this has led to a burgeoning market for liquid nutrients. Because of improper health claims, here, the FDA has been especially vigilant in monitoring advertising for these products.

early study in which it was demonstrated that certain *in vitro* interactions of common-form thiamin with selected dietary constituents in high fiber diet regimes, could influence thiamin bioavailability.

(b) Vitamin B6

Pyridoxal-5-phosphate (**PLP or P-5-P**) is considered the most metabolically active coenzyme and supplement of **vitamin B6**, and the most bioavailable form of this vitamin. This is due to the fact that P-5-P does not require prior activation by the liver to become functional, as is usual with **pyridoxine**, but is ready to perform its duties immediately following ingestion. P-5-P's bioavailability is enhanced when taken sublingually, which permits the active agent to enter the blood stream faster.

(c) Vitamin B12

For somewhat similar reasons the more neurologically active form of **B12**—methylcobalamin or **methyl B12**—has bioavailability superior to **cyanocobalamin**, the more common form. Typically the liver converts a small amount of cyanocobalamin into methylcobalamin. This latter form, together with adenosylcobalamin, represents the only active states of vitamin B12; all cobalamin must be converted into these states prior to the body's use. Consequently when methylcobalamin is directly administered to the body, the liver's task is made easier and the vitamin becomes more immediately available to the tissues. (In addition, human urinary excretion of methylcobalamin is said to be about one-third that of a similar dose of cyanocobalamin, indicating substantially greater tissue retention.) As with P-5-P, bioavailability is improved further when methylcobalamin is administered sublingually.

(d) Vitamin E

The most active form of vitamin E is **alpha-tocopherol.** Again the liver is implicated in this activity. In humans, all vitamin E forms are absorbed in the intestine. The majority of the absorbed vitamin E is then delivered to the liver, where the alpha-tocopherol is preferentially secreted into the blood circulation for delivery to tissues. This preference has to do with the number and position of methyl (i.e., CH_3) groups in the molecule; alpha-tocopherol's superior bioactivity is because it is more widely distributed than the other forms—beta-, delta-, and gamma-tocopherols—on the chromanol molecular ring. Now to say it another way. . . . no, I guess that's enough.

(e) Minerals

Absorption rates and bioavailabilities of minerals depend on several factors, including pH (the degree of acidity or alkalinity), the mineral source and other food components being ingested at the same time, as well as the presence of other minerals.[9] It is also believed that the body's need for a mineral can affect its absorption, which

---

[9] Some minerals compete with each other for absorption by the body. A high intake of one might produce a deficiency of another mineral. Copper, iron, and zinc are examples of minerals with this competitive quality. Calcium and magnesium compete for absorption in the small intestine, and excessive amounts of either one will inhibit the absorption of the other.

is said to increase as the need increases. (For example, women—who need to replenish iron lost in menstruation—absorb a greater percentage of iron as compared to men.)

Following is an excerpt from an article that Dr. Linda Harvey of the Institute of Food Research, in Colney, Norwich, England, kindly sent me in manuscript form on the subject of mineral absorption and bioavailability. (The article was ultimately published in *Nutrition and Food Science* (2001; 31 (4): 179–82.):

> The bioavailability of a mineral is generally defined as a measure of the proportion of the total in a food, meal or diet that is utilized for normal body functions. For most minerals the amount that is absorbed from the gastrointestinal (GI) tract is the major determinant of bioavailability but this varies greatly among minerals. Absorption is affected by a range of factors including interactions with other dietary components in the gastrointestinal tract e.g., vitamin C increases iron absorption, whilst tannins have an inhibitory effect. In addition to these diet-related factors, there is also a range of host-related factors that affect absorption. These include the expression of cellular transporters, which carry the mineral from the gastric lumen into the bloodstream. Mineral absorption consists of three components; uptake from the gastrointestinal tract into the mucosal cells, transfer within the cells, and transport across the serosal transport into the circulation.

A few nutritionists insist that chelated mineral forms such as aspartates, picolinates, citrates, and glycinates are better utilized and absorbed than inorganic salts such as carbonates, oxides, and sulfates. (The chelation process binds a mineral to both the oxygen and the nitrogen of another molecule called a ligand.) However, some studies report no absorption difference between these forms though almost all would recognize the superior absorbability of the **picolinates**.

Timothy C. Birdsall, N.D., points out that picolinic acid is a natural product of metabolism in the body. He theorizes in his paper, "Zinc Picolinate: Absorption and Supplementation,"[10] that **zinc picolinate** is absorbed to a higher degree than other zinc supplements because use of exogenous zinc picolinate may uniquely provide the actual compound normally created by the body in the intestinal tract to facilitate absorption.[11] This may also be the reason why **chromium picolinate** is generally considered to be more bioavailable than chromium chloride. As noted in the discussion of that mineral, however, safety issues have been raised as to its use. (I found no particular safety issue as to the use of zinc picolinate.)

Beyond these various *preferred* forms of nutrients—preferred because of their molecular structure—there are supplement manufacturers who have added special "enhancements" they claim make their vitamins, etc., more bioavailable than competitive offerings. This brings up the matter of **"natural"** versus **"synthetic"** nutrients.

---

[10] *Alternative Medicine Review* (1996; 1:26–30).
[11] Dr. Gary W. Evans at the USDA Human Nutrition Laboratory in Grand Forks, N.D., earlier had put it this way: "Since our bodies utilize picolinic acid to absorb and transport certain minerals, and our cells recognize mineral picolinates and readily use them, it makes sense to design mineral supplements based on this knowledge."

(f) Natural or Synthetic

Not surprisingly, any seller who can find some peg to hang the word "natural" on to its product when advertising will do so. (One diligent researcher, though, claims he did a computer search of all of the 7 million clinical studies reported at Medline using the two terms and found only 13 dual references. He maintains that no conclusion can be drawn from these as to whether one type is better that the other. I decided not to repeat his effort.)

To start with, there is often confusion in terms. There are no definitive regulations governing the use of the word "natural" so vitamin C made from sugar, for example, which was made in turn from beet or corn sugar, can be called "natural" because it had its beginnings in natural sources: beets and corn. (Most commercial vitamin C is made from this process.) Synthetic vitamins, on the other hand, can be made from **any source**. In fact many of them are manufactured from coal tar derivatives.

To further add to the confusion, many of the so-called natural nutrients have synthetics added to increase potency, or to standardize the amount in a capsule or batch. In addition a salt form is often added to increase stability—e.g., acetate, chloride, or nitrate. Just take a look at the label on one or two of your vitamin bottles.

There seem to be, though, some benefits for nutrients that are more *clearly* natural. The sources from which these more natural nutrients are derived often contain **co-factors** that come with the nutrients in nature. For instance, some co-factors that are usually found with vitamin C are various **bioflavonoids,** which are pigment substances found in plants with excellent antioxidant characteristics and would be lacking in plain ascorbic acid. Man-made synthetic supplements may be a combination of some of the separate factors but under that view they are never the whole complex of synergistic factors found in nature. Many professionals believe that the "unknown" co-factors found in natural vitamins, not found in synthetic forms, act as catalysts which make the vitamins more effective (but see the earlier discussion of vitamin C for a contrary view).

One vitamin where there appears to be little controversy that the natural form is superior to the synthetic is **vitamin E**, as noted above in the discussion on that nutrient. Identified as "d-alpha tocopherol," this form is considered as much as twice as potent as the synthetic, labeled "dl-alpha tocopherol." That conclusion seems to have been validated in a study in 1998 of 10 subjects who were either given the natural or the synthetic form, with blood measurements taken at the end of the study. The principal investigator reported the two forms "are absorbed equally well through the gut, but the liver clearly prefers the natural form, transferring it to lipoproteins to be transported through the blood for deposition into the tissues." [12]

Before leaving the subject of bioavailability I should mention that many of these more absorbable, bioavailable forms will not be found in most drug stores. For example, if you are looking for the P-5-P form of vitamin B6,

---

[12] *American Journal of Clinical Nutrition* (April 1998; 67: 669–84).

you will probably need to go to a health food store. One benefit of dealing with those retailers is that products they carry often minimize the use of sugars, artificial colors, and miscellaneous substances that hold the nutrients together.

When to Take

Most vitamins and minerals should be **taken with food** to enhance their absorption, according to nutritionists. This is particularly true as to the fat-soluble vitamins such as A and E, as well as the omega-3s such as fish oil and the omega-6s such as evening primrose oil. (A few bites are said to suffice. Protein, though, will help mineral absorption.[13]) The exceptions here are amino acids, which most nutritionists suggest should be taken at least 30 minutes before any other food. That is because they compete with the amino acids found naturally in food. (The only amino acid discussed in this book is acetyl-l-carnitine, or ALC. Two others that were discussed in *Toes and Soles* were N-acetyl cysteine, NAC, and S-adenosylmethione, SAMe. As I mentioned before, there was not enough scientific evidence of their efficacy to warrant inclusion here in my estimation.)

Vitamin C can be taken with or without food. Be sure to take plenty of water with it; that is helpful with respect

---

[13] Some nutritionists suggest that if you take fiber supplements, you should wait a few hours before taking other supplements because the fiber can bind minerals and make them unavailable for the body to use.

to any supplement in order to avoid leaving residue in the esophagus.

It is preferable to spread supplement ingestion over the day. This is particularly true if you are taking large quantities of a nutrient such as vitamin C. One thing to remember in taking your nutrients is that whatever schedule you are on, try and maintain it consistently.

In the end, if your schedule gets discombobulated with all of this, take heart! Julie Garden-Robinson, Food and Nutrition Specialist at the North Dakota State University, says that even if you take supplements at the "wrong time," absorption only drops by 5 to 10 %.

Laying Out A Program

Based on the studies and other material in this book, I think the following supplement program would be a good one for most of us. The stated amounts are intended for daily use:

1. A vitamin B 50 complex capsule which provides a combination of all the B vitamins in 50 mg strengths, including biotin, choline, and inositol (except, of course, vitamin B12 where the amount might be 50 *mcg*, and folic acid, which might be around 400 *mcg*).
2. 200 mg *additional* B1. Personally I would use one of the more conventional forms such as thiamin mononitrate rather than allithiamine which may have superior bioavailability but costs about five

times as much. If cost is not a major concern, you might go for the allithiamine—still 200 mgs.

3. 1000 mcg (1 mg) *additional* B12 in the form of sublingual methylcobalamin—the superior bioavailable form of this nutrient.

4. 1000 mg (1 g) of vitamin C, perhaps as calcium ascorbate with flavenoids or rose hips added. Also people who already have too much stomach acid may find a buffered form of vitamin C to be preferable.

5. 400 IU of vitamin E in the natural d-alpha tocopherol form.

6. 200 mg of magnesium chelate.

7. 50 mg of zinc picolinate (as discussed earlier, this form is produced by bonding picolinic acid with the metal, resulting in a more absorbable, bioavailable product), with supplemental copper if possible.

The cost at retail for the foregoing 7 vitamins and minerals (disregarding the more expensive form of B1) would probably be somewhere around $1.55–1.65 per day, depending on where you shop, quantities purchased, etc. It becomes more expensive as we begin to add the following supplements from chapter 4:

8. 600 mg of alpha-lipoic acid or ALA.

9. 4000 mg (4 g) of evening primrose oil, to yield about 3400 mg of omega-6 EFAs, including about 400 mg of GLA.

10. 4000 mg (4 g) of fish oil, to yield about 3600 mg of omega-3 EFAs, including perhaps 2000 mg of EPA

and 800 mg of DHA, the balance being other EFAs.

11. 1000 mg of acetyl-l-carnitine or ALC.

There appears to be a wide retail price range for these last 4—anywhere from $3.75 to nearly twice that per day. A program involving all 11 of these nutrient supplements in the dosages indicated, however, is not one that needs to be slavishly followed to derive good value from supplementation. For example, the most costly, acetyl-l-carnitine, could be dropped fairly easily, in my opinion. This would reduce your outlay for these last 4 supplements by about a third. If you were intent on doing more chopping, you could perhaps cut the alpha-lipoic acid and the fish oil by half and the evening primrose all the way back to 1000 mg daily. In any event I think you should keep the first seven—the vitamin and mineral supplements—just as listed because of the synergy from their combined usage.

If you are careful, it certainly should be possible to get on a decent, effective nutrient supplementation program that would cost you $100 or so per month. Compare this, for example, with the monthly expense of taking typically prescribed dosages of Neurontin, which is the most frequently used medication for the pain of peripheral neuropathy. According to an article by Sharon See, Pharm.D., and Denise L. Balog, Pharm.D., "The Pharmacologic Management of Painful Diabetic Peripheral Neuropathy," the monthly cost for the "usual total daily dosage" of that drug —900 to 1800 mg—is $96.60 to $193.20.[14] (Indeed, some people spend much more than this for PN medications!)

And not only might using supplements regularly be

less expensive than relying solely on medication for symptomatic relief,[15] there is as mentioned at the very beginning of this book at least the possibility of **sustained neurological improvement.** With medications such as Neurontin there is only the possibility of dosage-related **pain relief**—offset by frequent side effects.

If you consider the dosages used in the clinical studies reported in this book, you will find the program outlined above to be rather conservative, even at the full dosages indicated. Please keep in mind, though, that it is based on my own assessment and weighing of the relative merits of all the nutrients discussed here. It might be a good idea to review whatever you intend to do with a qualified medical professional familiar with your medical history before starting out.

Finally understand, when you begin your new supplement regime you should not expect instant improvement. It will generally take three or four months before benefits will be realized to any noticeable extent.

---

[14] *Toes and Soles* reported that typical prices for typical doses of Neurontin—900 to 1200 mg daily—ran about $3.24 to $4.32 per day (see p. 58 in that book for a table of other medication costs).

[15] You might still need medication with your supplements but you should be able to cut back if your experience is anything like mine. As I said before, I still take Neurontin, but not as much as I used to and, more importantly, I have nowhere near the pain I had before. Talk to your doctor about your own situation.

End Note

In the last three years—ever since doing the research and writing my first book on peripheral neuropathy, *Numb Toes and Aching Soles*—I have talked with hundreds of PNers about steps they took for diagnosis and treatment. Some of them (maybe even you) have spent many months and many thousands of dollars looking for help. I cannot tell you the number of times these PNers reported having heard something such as the following from a doctor: "Mr. (or Mrs. or Miss) Whoever-you-are, the tests we ran on you have told us nothing concerning the cause of your neuropathy, and I am afraid there is really nothing medicine can do for you except perhaps provide a little pain relief."

In my opinion the best thing most of those PNers who got that message could have done was to have grabbed their hats, gone home and begun a sensible program of **nutrient supplementation**. I hope this book will prompt you to do the same, and that you will combine an **exercise program** with it that is comfortable and beneficial for you.

There are a couple of other important actions to take: join a neuropathy support group, if you have not already done so, in order that you may share experiences with others in the same boat. (See if you can find one in your area by calling the Neuropathy Association at 1-800-247-6968.) Also, to the extent you are able, take on some new project or activity to get your mind off your PNishness (writing these books, for example, has helped me as much as anything). To parody an old real estate saying: participate, participate, participate! It will make you feel better.

(Please note that following the index, there is a book order form.)

Council for Responsible Nutrition

Vitamins: Comparison of current RDIs, new DRIs and ULs

Vitamin	Current RDI*	New DRI**	UL***
Vitamin A	5000 IU (3000 IU)	900 mcg (10,000 IU)	3000 mcg
Vitamin C	60 mg	90 mg	2000 mg
Vitamin D	400 IU (10 mcg)	15 mcg (600 IU)	50 mcg (2000 IU)
Vitamin E	30 IU (20 mg)	15 mg#	1000 mg
Vitamin K	80 mcg	120 mcg	ND
Thiamin	1.5 mg	1.2 mg	ND
Riboflavin	1.7 mg	1.3 mg	ND
Niacin	20 mg	16 mg	35 mg
Vitamin B-6	2 mg	1.7 mg	100 mg
Folate	400 mcg (0.4 mg)	400 mcg from food, 200 mcg synthetic##	1000 mcg synthetic
Vitamin B-12	6 mcg	2.4 mcg###	ND
Biotin	300 mcg	30 mcg	ND
Pantothenic acid	10 mg	5 mg	ND
Choline	Not established	550 mg	3500 mg

*The Reference Daily Intake (RDI) is the value established by the Food and Drug Administration (FDA) for use in nutrition labeling. It was based initially on the highest 1968 Recommended Dietary Allowance (RDA) for each nutrient, to assure that needs were met for all age groups.

**The Dietary Reference Intakes (DRI) are the most recent set of dietary recommendations established by the Food and Nutrition Board of the Institute of Medicine, 1997–2001. They replace previous RDAs, and may be the basis for eventually updating the RDIs. The value shown here is the highest DRI for each nutrient.

***The upper limit (UL) is the upper level of intake considered to be **safe** for use by adults, incorporating a safety factor. In some cases, lower ULs have been established for children.

#Historical vitamin E conversion factors were amended in the DRI report, so that 15 mg is defined as the equivalent of 22 IU of natural vitamin E or 33 IU of synthetic vitamin E.

##It is recommended that women of childbearing age obtain 400 mcg of synthetic folic acid from fortified breakfast cereals or dietary supplements, in addition to dietary folate.

###It is recommended that people over 50 meet the B-12 recommendation through fortified foods or supplements, to improve bioavailability.

ND Upper Limit not determined. No adverse effects observed from high intakes of the nutrient.

Council for Responsible Nutrition, 2001
1875 Eye Street N.W. Suite 400, Washington, D.C. 20006 • (202) 872-1488

Council for Responsible Nutrition

Minerals: Comparison of current RDIs, new DRIs and ULs

Mineral	Current RDI*	New DRI**	UL***
Calcium	1000 mg	1300 mg	2500 mg
Iron	18 mg	18 mg	45 mg
Phosphorus	1000 mg	1250 mg	4000 mg
Iodine	150 mcg	150 mcg	1100 mcg
Magnesium	400 mg	420 mg	350 mg#
Zinc	15 mg	11 mg	40 mg
Selenium	70 mcg	55 mcg	400 mcg
Copper	2 mg	0.9 mg	10 mg
Manganese	2 mg	2.3 mg	11 mg
Chromium	120 mcg	35 mcg	ND
Molybdenum	75 mcg	45 mcg	2000 mcg

*The Reference Daily Intake (RDI) is the value established by the Food and Drug Administration (FDA) for use in nutrition labeling. It was based initially on the highest 1968 Recommended Dietary Allowance (RDA) for each nutrient, to assure that needs were met for all age groups.

**The Dietary Reference Intakes (DRI) are the most recent set of dietary recommendations established by the Food and Nutrition Board of the Institute of Medicine, 1997–2001. They replace previous RDAs, and may be the basis for eventually updating the RDIs. The value shown here is the highest DRI for each nutrient.

***The upper limit (UL) is the upper level of intake considered to be **safe** for use by adults, incorporating a safety factor. In some cases, lower ULs have been established for children.

#Upper limit for magnesium applies only to intakes from dietary supplements or pharmaceutical products, not including intakes from food and water.

ND Upper Limit not determined. No adverse effects observed from high intakes of the nutrient.

Council for Responsible Nutrition, 2001
1875 Eye Street N.W. Suite 400, Washington, D.C. 20006 • (202) 872-1488

Council for Responsible Nutrition

Vitamins: Historical Comparison of RDIs, RDAs and DRIs, 1968 to Present

Vitamin	RDI*	RDA**	1968 RDA**	1974 RDA**	1980 RDA**	1989 DRIs***
Vitamin A	5000 IU	5000 IU	1000 RE (5000 IU)	1000 RE	1000 RE (3000 IU)	900 mcg
Vitamin C	60 mg	60 mg	45 mg	60 mg	60 mg	90 mg
Vitamin D	400 IU (10 mcg)	400 IU (10 mcg)	400 IU (10 mcg)	10 mcg (400 IU)	10 mcg (400 IU)	15 mcg (600 IU)
Vitamin E	30 IU (20 mg)	30 IU (20 mg)	15 IU (10 mg)	10 mg (15 IU)	10 mg (15 IU)	15 mg[#]
Vitamin K	80 mcg	—	—	70–140 mcg	80 mcg	120 mcg
Thiamin	1.5 mg	1.5 mg	1.5 mg	1.5 mg	1.5 mg	1.2 mg
Riboflavin	1.7 mg	1.7 mg	1.8 mg	1.7 mg	1.8 mg	1.3 mg
Niacin	20 mg	20 mg	20 mg	19 mg	20 mg	16 mg
Vitamin B-6	2 mg	2 mg	2 mg	2.2 mg	2 mg	1.7 mg
Folate	0.4 mg (400 mcg)	400 mcg	400 mcg	400 mcg	200 mcg	400 mcg food, 200 mcg synthetic[##]
Vitamin B-12	6 mcg	6 mcg	3 mcg	3 mcg	2 mcg	2.4 mcg[###]
Biotin	(300 mcg)	150–300 mcg	100–300 mcg	100–200 mcg	30–100 mcg	30 mcg
Pantothenic acid	10 mg	5–10 mg	5–10 mg	4–7 mg	4–7 mg	5 mg
Choline	—	—	—	—	—	550 mg

*The Reference Daily Intake (RDI) is the value established by the Food and Drug Administration (FDA) for use in nutrition labeling. It was based initially on the highest 1968 Recommended Dietary Allowance (RDA) for each nutrient, to assure that needs were met for all age groups.

**The RDAs were established and periodically revised by the Food and Nutrition Board. Value shown is the highest RDA for each nutrient, in the year indicated for each revision.

***The Dietary Reference Intakes (DRI) are the most recent set of dietary recommendations established by the Food and Nutrition Board of the Institute of Medicine, 1997–2001. They replace previous RDAs, and may be the basis for eventually updating the RDIs. The value shown here is the highest DRI for each nutrient.

[#]Historical vitamin E conversion factors were amended in the DRI report, so that 15 mg is defined as the equivalent of 22 IU of natural vitamin E or 33 IU of synthetic vitamin E.

[##]It is recommended that women of childbearing age obtain 400 mcg of synthetic folic acid from fortified breakfast cereals or dietary supplements, in addition to dietary folate.

[###]It is recommended that people over 50 meet the B-12 recommendation through fortified foods or supplements, to improve bioavailability.

Council for Responsible Nutrition, 2001
1875 Eye Street N.W. Suite 400, Washington, D.C. 20006 • (202) 872-1488

158

Minerals: Historical Comparison of RDIs, RDAs and DRIs, 1968 to Present

Nutrient	RDI*	1968 RDA**	1974 RDA**	1980 RDA**	1989 RDA**	DRIs***
Calcium	1000 mg	1300 mg	1200 mg	1200 mg	1200 mg	1300 mg
Phosphorus	1000 mg	1300 mg	1200 mg	1200 mg	1200 mg	1250 mg (700 adult)
Iron	18 mg	18 mg	18 mg	18 mg	15 mg	18 mg
Iodine	150 mcg	150 mcg	150 mcg	150 mcg	150 mcg	150 mcg
Magnesium	400 mg	400 mg	400 mg	400 mg	400 mg	420 mg
Zinc	15 mg	10–15 mg	15 mg	15 mg	15 mg	11 mg
Selenium	70 mcg	—	—	—	70 mcg	55 mcg
Copper	2 mg	—	—	2–3 mg	1.5–3 mg	0.9 mg
Manganese	2 mg	—	2.5–7 mg	2.5–5 mg	2–5 mg	2.3 mg
Chromium	120 mcg	—	—	50–200 mcg	50–200 mcg	35 mcg
Molybdenum	75 mcg	—	45–500 mg	150–500 mcg	75–250 mcg	45 mcg

*The Reference Daily Intake (RDI) is the value established by the Food and Drug Administration (FDA) for use in nutrition labeling. It was based initially on the highest 1968 Recommended Dietary Allowance (RDA) for each nutrient, to assure that needs were met for all age groups.

**The RDAs were established and periodically revised by the Food and Nutrition Board. Value shown is the highest RDA for each nutrient, in the year indicated for each revision.

***The Dietary Reference Intakes (DRI) are the most recent set of dietary recommendations established by the Food and Nutrition Board of the Institute of Medicine, 1997–2001. They replace previous RDAs, and may be the basis for eventually updating the RDIs. The value shown here is the highest DRI for each nutrient.

Council for Responsible Nutrition, 2001
1875 Eye Street N.W. Suite 400, Washington, D.C. 20006 • (202) 872-1488

Index

Folic acid. *See* Folate/folic acid
Food and Drug Administration (FDA), 2, 131n50, 141n8
Food sources: of ALA (alpha-lipoic acid), 43; of ascorbic acid (vitamin C), 70, 106n2; of bioflavonoids, 73; of biotin, 58; of carnitine, 126; of chromium, 88, 90–91; of cobalamin (B12), 55–56, 56n47; of essential fatty acids (EFAs), 106, 106n2, 110; of essential nutrients generally, 24–25; of folate/folic acid, 60; of inositol, 62, 64; of lecithin, 66; of magnesium, 97; of myoinositol, 64; of niacin (B3), 41; of riboflavin (B2), 40; of selenium, 99; of thiamin (B1), 38; of vitamin E, 77, 106n2; of zinc, 102. *See also* specific foods
Food with nutrient supplements, 148–49
France, 8, 27n1, 70n69, 107–8
Free radicals, 39, 39n20, 59, 68, 70n69, 74, 74n73, 79, 98, 98n19, 117
Fruits, 62, 64, 70, 70n69, 73, 97. *See also* specific fruit

G (gram), 27
Gaby, Alan R., 36–37
Gaines Nutrition, 37
Gamma linolenic acid (GLA): and antioxidants, 113; ascorbyl-GLA, 112–13; daily program/dosage of, 150; and EFA balance, 114n22; food sources of, 106, 110–11; and side effects, 115; synergistic effect of alpha-lipoic acid and, 112, 119n28, 121; therapeutic dosages for, 114; for treatment of diabetes, 21n4, 90, 125; for treatment of peripheral neuropathy, xv, 68, 90, 112–13, 113n18; and vitamin C, 68
Gamma-tocopherol, 74n73
Garden-Robinson, Julie, 149
Garlic, 38, 99
Garlic oil, 38
Gastric surgery, 51n39
Gastritis, 3n3
Gastrointestinal problems, 64, 71–72, 115, 133, 139
GBLE (ginkgo biloba extract), 130
General nutrient supplementation, 15–17. *See also* specific nutrients
Germany, 8, 21, 33n11, 35, 42–43, 111–12, 117, 118, 118n25, 120–22
Gingivitis, 80
Ginkgo biloba, xv, 79, 128–31
Ginseng, 127
GJK (goshajinkigan), 131–33
GLA. *See* Gamma linolenic acid (GLA)
Glaucoma, 3n3
Glossitis, 80, 81
Glucose, xiii, 92, 116
Glucose intolerance, 21n4, 88–89

Glutathione, 39, 68, 106n2, 116, 116n23
Glutathione peroxidase, 97–98
Goshajinkigan (GJK), 131–33
Government support for nutrient studies, 8
Grains, 62, 64, 99, 102
Gram (g), 27
Grape seed extract, 127
Grapefruit, 62
Greece, 57
Green leafy vegetables, 40, 58, 60, 66, 77, 97, 106
Green tea, 127
Growth disorders, 99, 102

H2 blockers, 56, 99
H vitamin. *See* Vitamin H
Hair, 28, 32, 102, 115
Halibut, 106
Harvard Medical School, 4n4, 113
Harvey, Linda, 144
HCY (homocysteine), 28, 48–49, 48n32, 55, 59
Headaches, 93, 103n26, 115
Health food stores, 148
Hearing loss, 51n39, 83, 85
Heart attack, xv, 75, 113
Heart disease, 22, 22n5, 28, 47, 48, 51, 70n69, 75, 75n75, 80
Heart health, 75, 75n75, 121, 126
Heart rhythm, 93, 97, 121–22
Hemoglobin, 54n44, 106
Hemorrhage in brain, xv, 131
Hendler, Sheldon, 47
Heparin, 79, 115, 130
Herbs, xiv-xv, 6, 79, 127, 128–35
Herring, 106
Hexavalent chromium, 88n2
Higdon, Jane, 71–73
High blood pressure, 40, 93
HIV-positive people, 37, 41, 53, 94n13, 95–96, 98, 112, 124n40, 126
Homocysteine (HCY), 28, 48–49, 48n32, 55, 59
Hops flower, 127
Hormones, 105–6
Horsetail, 38
Houston Immunological Institute, 95
Hungary, 35
Huntington's chorea, 103n26
Hyperkinesia, 103n26
Hyperpigmentation, 80
Hypersomnolence, 103n26
Hypertension, 96
Hypochromic anemia, 80, 84
Hypoglycemic medications, 79
Hypokalemic paralysis, 103n26
Hypophosphatemia, 85

Idiopaths, 19
IF (intrinsic factor), 47

The *Numb Toes* Books

T his is the third in the *Numb Toes* series of books written by John Senneff dealing with peripheral neuropathy. Each of them is designed to give PN patients and their caretakers as much practical information as possible concerning this serious affliction. *Nutrients for Neuropathy* thoroughly covers an especially important treatment option—nutrient supplementation.

John Senneff's first book, *Numb Toes and Aching Soles: Coping with Peripheral Neuropathy*, published in July 1999 and in its 5th printing when this was written, is the much-acclaimed basic primer on PN. Sold all over the world and favorably reviewed in more than 70 medical and other journals and publications, it covers symptoms, causes, tests, and treatments—conventional as well as alternative. Day-to-day coping strategies are dealt with in depth. Its nearly 300 pages include comments from 12 leading neurologists and over 200 patient stories on pain and other treatment experiences.

The sequel, *Numb Toes and Other Woes: More on Peripheral Neuropathy,* came out in July 2001. Many new clinical findings on neuropathy therapies are detailed in its 250+ pages. Important medical treatments emerging from laboratories are exhaustively covered as well. Alternative treatment strategies for diabetic and other neuropathies are particularly emphasized.

All of these books may be ordered on the order form following this page or from your favorite book store. Please note the special combination prices available when an order form is used.

Information concerning *Numb Toes and Aching Soles* and *Numb Toes and Other Woes*, including detailed descriptions, excerpts, and reviews, may be found at our web site, www.medpress.com.

BOOK ORDER FORM

(Order extra copies for any friends or relatives you think might benefit—even for your doctor!)

Telephone orders: Call 1-888-MED-9898 toll free (1-888-633-9898).

Fax orders: Fax the form you have filled in below to 1-210-641-6334.

Postal orders: Mail the form you have filled in below to:
MedPress, P.O. Box 691546, San Antonio, TX 78269

Please send me the following:
Nutrients for Neuropathy
_____ copies (paperback), $19.95 each.
Numb Toes and Aching Soles: Coping with Peripheral Neuropathy
_____ copies (paperback edition), $22.95 each.
_____ copies (professional case bound edition), $29.95 each.
Numb Toes and Other Woes: More on Peripheral Neuropathy
_____ copies (paperback edition), $22.95 each.
_____ copies (professional case bound edition), $29.95 each.

(Special 10%-off combination offer: For ordering both *Numb Toes and Aching Soles* and *Numb Toes and Other Woes* in paperback, $41.30. For both in professional case bound, $53.90. If *Nutrients for Neuropathy* (paperback) is to be included, add $17.95 to total.

Shipping & Handling: Please add for U.S. deliveries, $5 for one book, $3 for each additional (outside the U.S., $8 for one book, $4 for each additional).
For special U.S. Priority mailing—usually 2 to 3 days, add $3.95 more for first book, $2 more for each additional.
Check here: _____.
For special Global Priority outside of U.S.—usually 4 to 5 days, add $9 more for first book, $4 more for each additional.
Check here: _____.

Sales Tax: For shipments to Texas addresses, please add 7.875% to the total (books plus S & H).

Payment: Check _____ Postal Money Order _____ Credit Card _____
Visa ___ Master Card _____ Am Ex _____ Discover _____

Card No.: _____ **Exp. Date:** ___/___

Name on Card: _____

Address: _____

_____

Tel. No.: _____

(Unless a priority service is chosen above, please allow 8 to 10 days for U. S. deliveries, 5 to 6 weeks for deliveries outside of U.S.)
Thank you!

ME
FIRST